Establishing a Research and Evaluation Capability for the Joint Medical Education and Training Campus

Sheila Nataraj Kirby, Julie A. Marsh, Harry J. Thie

Prepared for the Office of the Secretary of Defense

Approved for public release; distribution unlimited

Center for Military Health Policy Research

A JOINT ENDEAVOR OF RAND HEALTH AND THE
RAND NATIONAL DEFENSE RESEARCH INSTITUTE

The research reported here was sponsored by the Office of the Secretary of Defense (OSD). The research was conducted jointly by the Center for Military Health Policy Research, a RAND Health program, and the Forces and Resources Policy Center, a RAND National Defense Research Institute (NDRI) program. NDRI is a federally funded research and development center sponsored by OSD, the Joint Staff, the Unified Combatant Commands, the Navy, the Marine Corps, the defense agencies, and the defense Intelligence Community under Contract W74V8H-06-C-0002.

Library of Congress Library of Congress Control Number: 2011927969

ISBN: 978-0-8330-5064-9

Published 2011 by the RAND Corporation
1776 Main Street, P.O. Box 2138, Santa Monica, CA 90407-2138
1200 South Hayes Street, Arlington, VA 22202-5050
4570 Fifth Avenue, Suite 600, Pittsburgh, PA 15213-2665
RAND URL: http://www.rand.org/
To order RAND documents or to obtain additional information, contact
Distribution Services: Telephone: (310) 451-7002;
Fax: (310) 451-6915; Email: order@rand.org

Preface

Both the 2005 Base Realignment and Closure (BRAC) Commission and the 2006 Quadrennial Defense Review called for the transformation of medical education and training to foster interchangeability and interoperability among medical personnel and units across the services. The BRAC report recommended relocating basic and specialty enlisted medical training to Fort Sam Houston, Texas, to take advantage of economies of scale and the opportunity for joint training. To fulfill the BRAC recommendation, a joint medical education and training campus (METC) is being established at Fort Sam Houston.

The RAND Corporation was asked to provide technical and research assistance in several areas to facilitate implementation of joint medical training and education. One of the tasks was to examine the need for and feasibility of establishing a research and evaluation capability within METC akin to an office of institutional research (OIR, also variously called an office of institutional planning, institutional effectiveness, or institutional research and planning), typically found in higher-education institutions, or an evaluation office, typically found in entities whose mission is training. This monograph documents the results of that task. It makes a case for establishing an OIR within METC based on two long-term goals for the campus: (1) becoming a high-performing learning organization and (2) seeking accreditation as a community college rather than becoming accredited under the umbrella of the Community College of the Air Force. Achieving either or both of these goals requires METC to adopt a clear model of organizational improvement with well-defined metrics for measuring its performance and using research and evaluation to assess and improve that performance.

This monograph uses data from interviews with directors of OIRs at several four-year undergraduate institutions and community colleges to examine the scope and structure of typical OIRs. Given that METC's mission is narrower than that of a community college—it is focused on technical training, not on providing broader learning and education—the monograph examines lessons learned regarding research and evaluation activities in organizations with missions similar to METC's. These include corporate universities; the Defence Medical Education and Training Agency, METC's counterpart in the United Kingdom, which was established to provide joint medical education and training to the three military services in that country; and other federal agencies. Because these organizations emphasize the evaluation of training programs, the monograph also reviews the guidelines offered by the U.S. Government Accountability Office for assessing strategic training and development efforts in the federal government. This work should be of interest to personnel and military planners and educators involved in medical workforce education and training and those interested in organizational transformation.

This research was sponsored the Military Health System Office of Transformation and conducted jointly by RAND Health's Center for Military Health Policy Research and the Forces and Resources Policy Center of the RAND National Defense Research Institute (NDRI). The Center for Military Health Policy Research taps RAND expertise in both defense and health policy to conduct research for the Department of Defense, the Veterans Administration, and nonprofit organizations. RAND Health aims to transform the well-being of all people by solving complex problems in health and health care. NDRI is a federally funded research and development center sponsored by the Office of the Secretary of Defense, the Joint Staff, the Unified Combatant Commands, the Navy, the Marine Corps, the defense agencies, and the defense Intelligence Community.

For more information on the Center for Military Health Policy Research, see http://www.rand.org/multi/military/ or contact the co-directors (contact information is provided on the web page). For more information on the Forces and Resources Policy Center, see http://www.rand.org/nsrd/about/frp.html or contact the director (contact information is provided on the web page).

Contents

Figures

Tables

Summary

The 2005 Base Realignment and Closure (BRAC) Commission report recommended relocating basic and specialty enlisted medical training to Fort Sam Houston, Texas, to take advantage of economies of scale and facilitate the opportunity for joint training. To fulfill the BRAC recommendation, a joint medical education and training campus (METC) was established at Fort Sam Houston and became officially operational on June 30, 2010, although its initial training course, Radiography Specialist, began in April. Other courses will be phased in over several months. METC will consolidate most of the medical enlisted training currently being conducted at several military installations at Fort Sam Houston. When it is fully established, it will be responsible for training more than 100 enlisted medical specialties and will be one of the world's largest medical education and training institutions, with an annual throughput of more than 24,500 students, an average daily student load of more than 8,000, and a total of 1,400 faculty and staff members. The vision is for METC to become the nation's leading military medical education and training institution and its stated goals are to capture best practices and achieve efficiencies in training and to transform itself into a high-performing, "learning" organization.

RAND was asked to provide technical and research assistance in several areas related to METC's implementation, including the need for and feasibility of establishing a research and evaluation capability within METC—the focus of this monograph.

The study aimed to address two major research questions:

1.   Does METC need a research and evaluation capability?
2.   What lessons can be learned from institutions with missions similar to that of METC in terms of research and evaluation activities and the structure and scope of an office of institutional research (OIR)?

We discuss each of these issues in turn, providing a description of our data, approach, and findings.

Does METC Need a Research and Evaluation Capability?

To answer this question, we took as a starting point METC's avowed long-term goals of becoming a high-performing organization and seeking accreditation. To understand the role that research and evaluation play in high-performing organizations, we examined the literature on high-performing organizations and models of organizational improvement that such organizations typically implement. We focused on the framework established by the Malcolm Baldrige National Quality Award (MBNQA) program, both because it is arguably the nation's most prestigious quality award and because it has been adapted for the education sector. We reviewed the process and requirements for accreditation at three institutional accrediting bodies—the Southern Association of Colleges and Schools, the Council on Occupational Education, and the Accrediting Bureau of Health Education Schools—whose missions seem best aligned with METC's proposed purpose and structure.

Characteristics of a High-Performing Organization

Our review showed that high-performing organizations are focused on achieving results and outcomes and that, "to sustain a focus on results, high-performing organizations continuously assess and benchmark performance and efforts to improve performance" (GAO, 2004b, p. 7). At the heart of most high-performing organizations is an organizational improvement model or methodology, such as Total Quality

Management, Lean Production, Six Sigma, and the MBNQA framework. All these models emphasize measurement and analysis of organizational performance and the use of these results for organizational improvement. Thus, to support its goal of becoming a high-performing organization, METC will need to develop and sustain the capability to collect, organize, analyze, and use data on a variety of processes and outcomes to support innovation and performance excellence. In addition, it will need to review these indicators and its data and analysis systems on a periodic basis to adapt to new or changing environments and stakeholder needs.

Requirements for Accreditation

In the United States, accreditation is the primary stamp of approval indicating that an institution provides a legitimate education that meets standards of quality. Individual programs in an institution may also be accredited, which serves as an indicator that an educational program has met specific quality standards. Many of METC's programs require program accreditation. Early on in planning, it was discussed that METC may one day seek formal accreditation as a degree-granting institution of higher education, accessible to members of all services.

Accreditation bodies are increasingly requiring programs and institutions to develop and implement quality-improvement plans and learning objectives and to provide credible evidence of the value added to student learning and subsequent workforce outcomes. The standards of the three accrediting organizations that we examined in detail also specify a variety of quality indicators that may be used for assessment and evaluation of occupational education programs, including (among others) graduation or completion rate, employment or placement rate, pass rate on professional licensure exams, employer satisfaction, participant satisfaction, and assessment of occupational skills and knowledge. Notably, several of these indicators (e.g., licensure exam pass rate, employer satisfaction, placement rate) require follow-up with program graduates and supervisors. In addition, several organizations provide benchmarks for certain indicators (such as graduation rates or licensure exam pass rates), typically determined by evaluating data from current organizational members or peer institutions.

While standards for all three organizations are relatively non-prescriptive, a handful of standards may present larger substantive issues for METC, in particular those related to governance structures, program length, and faculty credentials. Regardless, should METC seek accreditation in the future, it will need a research and evaluation capability to meet the accreditation requirement for institutional improvement plans, embedded assessment, and tracking of a variety of indicators.

What Lessons Can Be Learned from Institutions with Similar Missions?

To gather lessons learned from institutions with similar missions, we undertook three research tasks.

First, because METC is akin to a technical community college, we conducted a series of interviews with the heads of OIRs at nine selected colleges (chosen because they were large and more likely to adopt best practices or were widely regarded as exemplars) and representatives from four professional associations and networks with which these leaders were affiliated.

Second, because METC's mission is more limited than that of a traditional college (in the sense that it will offer primarily technical training, rather than general education), we examined research and evaluation activities in organizations with missions similar to METC's, including

- corporate universities
- METC's counterpart in the United Kingdom, the Defence Medical Education and Training Agency (DMETA), which was established by the UK Ministry of Defence in 2003 to provide joint education and training for military medical personnel in the three services (British Army, Royal Navy, and Royal Air Force)
- other federal agencies, such as the Veterans Health Administration (VHA), that invest considerable resources in training and development.

We reviewed extant literature on corporate universities. Because DMETA is closely allied with METC in terms of mission and focus, we conducted interviews with senior leaders there and reviewed materials that they provided. To understand what federal agencies were doing, we reviewed extensive work done by the U.S. Government Accountability Office (GAO) in this area. As part of the larger RAND project, we had conducted interviews with several senior leaders at the VHA. In those interviews, we also gathered information on that organization's approach to research and evaluation, which we report here.

Third, because all these organizations emphasize evaluation of training programs, we reviewed the strategic framework outlined by the GAO for designing and implementing training evaluations. This process incorporated best practices and offered several useful guidelines for METC in terms of undertaking evaluations of training programs.

Insights from Community Colleges and Four-Year Institutions

OIRs in higher-education institutions appear to have a range of functions: data management, internal reporting, external reporting, accreditation, and strategic planning, to name a few. In particular, respondents stressed the importance of organizing data collection and management, delineating a common terminology and data definitions, and establishing a centralized data warehouse. The majority of institutions reported conducting periodic surveys of students, including entry and exit surveys, student satisfaction surveys, and course evaluations. A few institutions (generally the four-year colleges and larger community colleges) reported participating in research and evaluations of programs or initiatives. These evaluations were often internal and were intended to inform policy review and improvements. Respondents also offered various lessons learned regarding the structure and governance of an OIR. (See the section "Recommendations for METC," later in the Summary, for additional details.)

Insights from Corporate Universities

Corporate universities are separate entities that are primarily responsible for the development and implementation of training programs for members of the parent organization (Meister, 1994). METC closely resembles a corporate university in that it was set up to provide consolidated medical education and training to Army, Navy, and Air Force medical enlisted personnel to support the mission of the Military Health System (MHS). Our review of the literature revealed some common themes. First, although corporate universities differ in scope and function, measurement and evaluation of program effectiveness is always a key component, and corporate training leaders devote significant resources and attention to evaluation. Second, numerous authors noted that best-practice organizations build evaluation into training programs early by devoting considerable attention to evaluation issues in the program development and planning phase. Third, best-practice organizations focus on the customer in their evaluation efforts. Evaluators in these corporations consult with customers—broadly construed—to determine their requirements, which standards to set, and which outcomes to measure (Dixon, 1996). Fourth, evaluation in best-practice organizations is focused not simply on program improvement but on broader organizational improvement as well. Thus, evaluations are designed and implemented with strategic organizational goals in mind.

Insights from the Defence Medical Education and Training Agency

While DMETA provides training to a broad array of military medical personnel, both officers and enlisted, it is similar to METC in that it provides training to allied health professionals (e.g., radiographers, operating department technicians) and combat medical technicians or medical assistants. DMETA's approach to training is guided by the Defence Systems Approach to Training model, which espouses a cyclical but iterative approach to training and emphasizes continuous evaluation throughout the process to allow adjustments to be made as and when needed.

All training is evaluated at DMETA. Internally, it is expected to measure through an after-action review an individual's immediate outcomes and the learning transfer achieved by the training activity. In addition, the services are expected to validate changes in the behavior of the individual as a result of the training activity and how well the enhancement of knowledge, skills, or attitudes has prepared an individual for his or her role, as well as the contribution of training to the achievement of business or operational goals. However, DMETA has taken a more proactive stance in coordinating the external valida- tion across the UK's three military services, implementing an "early- warning feedback" form of external validation to identify and inform the requirement for a more rigorous and full evaluation of the training. The results of this full evaluation are fed into the system and used to check the accuracy of job performance requirements and to prove that the training being delivered still meets the operational requirements of the services.

In addition, DMETA must collect data and report annually on several performance indicators that are part of the Defence Balanced Scorecard. These indicators include, among others, the percentage of DMETA personnel who achieved the mandatory individual military training; the extent to which provision of initial and career, profes- sional, and continuation training meet the requirements, standards, and timescales of the services; and whether the customer confidence index score is within the set target.

Insights from Federal Agencies

In 2004, the GAO reported on several federal agencies' experiences and lessons learned regarding designing effective training and development programs. It noted that (1) evaluation of training was a key component of the training process at the organizations studied, and (2) the agen- cies had begun to use more comprehensive and sophisticated techniques for assessing the extent to which training and development programs increased employees' knowledge and skills and enhanced individual and organizational performance. These techniques included pre- and post-testing, tracking changes in individual and program performance, and some limited use of return-on-investment analyses. Our case study of the VHA (see Kirby et al., 2010) showed that over the last several years, the VHA has spent considerable time and effort transform- ing itself into a high-performing learning organization, leveraging its National Center for Organizational Development, a central office that measures and monitors the organizational health of the VHA. In addi- tion, it has strongly embraced continuous assessment, feedback, and redesign for the entire organization's training and development programs and invested considerable resources in evaluation, performance measurement, and metrics for organizational improvement.

GAO's strategic framework for designing and implementing effective training and development programs, discussed in Chapter Five of this monograph, highlights the importance of integrating evaluation into each step of the training and development process because agencies need to be able to demonstrate how these efforts help develop employees and improve the agencies' performance. We also review various types and levels of evaluation.

Recommendations for METC

There is a clear need for a research and evaluation capability within METC that can further its current goal of becoming a high-performing organization and its future goal of being accredited. Such a capability can also help address the federal government's increasing need to measure performance and cost-effectiveness and to provide evidence of the value added by training. At community colleges, such a research and evaluation capability is typically housed in an OIR, and this requires defining the structure and scope of such an office. Our interviews and literature reviews point to some useful recommendations in this regard.

Structure, Governance, and Staffing

In terms of structure, governance, and staffing, METC would benefit from the following guidance in establishing its OIR:

- Position the METC OIR so that it reports to senior leadership and its director is part of the senior management team. This arrangement would help ensure that the office is taken seriously and that the director has credibility and the authority to access the needed data.
- Ensure that the office is adequately staffed and that the staff have a mix of skills, including technical skills (e.g., statistics, information technology, programming), as well as broader enter-

prise knowledge and communication and interpersonal skills—particularly the ability to convey the meaning of the data collected on the training and development activities. Staffing in OIRs in the larger community colleges and four-year institutions tended to range from four to 14 full-time staff members; size is obviously a function of the scope of the office.

- Collaborate with other METC departments, participate in institutional committees, and extend opportunities for all concerned stakeholders to provide input into the continuous improvement process and gain buy-in.
- Encourage OIR staff to participate in professional associations and networks to learn about best practices and to foster personal and professional growth. In addition, ensure that the OIR director develops collaborative relationships with community colleges, corporate universities, other federal agencies (such as the VHA), and DMETA to learn about best practices in research and evaluation activities.

OIR Scope

In terms of scope, the following recommendations were relevant to METC's mission:

- Examine METC's vision and goals and map them against the types of data needed to measure progress. Then, examine the institutional structure within METC to delineate the roles and responsibilities of the various offices to avoid both duplication of effort and the overlooking of essential functions.
- Consider the following, among other functions, when defining the scope of the OIR:
  - Build a centralized data warehouse to track students, indicators of student learning, and student progress.
  - Work with the leadership team to collect and report data for METC's balanced scorecard and help translate the results so that they can be used for organizational improvement.
  - Collect, analyze, and report basic data on the institution that might be needed for external reporting.

- Design and evaluate training programs:
  - o Work with other academic offices responsible for the design and implementation of training to incorporate evaluation from the office's inception.
  - o Examine the full gamut of training programs, and determine the types of evaluations that might be appropriate for each. Generally accepted models of evaluation have several stages that involve increasingly more complex and expensive measures. The office could help determine which programs would warrant the higher and more complex levels of evaluation that would require following up with supervisors and others in the field to determine the impact on performance.
  - o Communicate and disseminate results in ways that allow them to be used to improve training.
- Work with program accreditation committees to understand the types of data and reporting required, and ensure that they are feasible.

The roles and responsibilities of the OIR are likely to change as it matures, but it is important to lay the groundwork now and to ensure that these functions are housed somewhere within METC, either in the OIR or in other offices. Perhaps the most immediate and important of these functions is to be proactive in designing a centralized warehouse for data with carefully defined, consistent data elements and data sources, clearly identifying the rationale and responsibility for data collection. The database should be designed to be flexible and adaptable so that it can easily respond to changing and additional demands as METC becomes more established and as the scope of the OIR expands. Recognizing the centrality of research and evaluation activities by establishing an OIR under the direction of an experienced institutional researcher is an important first step to becoming a high-performing, results-driven organization.

Acknowledgments

This study was sponsored by the flag officer steering committee and the executive integrated process team overseeing establishment of the joint METC at Fort Sam Houston, Texas, as part of the transformation of the MHS mandated by the Quadrennial Defense Review. Both the steering committee and the executive integrated process team include senior representatives from each service, the Joint Staff, and U.S. Joint Forces Command. We are grateful to them for their guidance and support of the study.

We owe a debt of gratitude to our many respondents, without whose generous assistance the study could not have been completed. In particular, we are grateful to the senior leaders of DMETA in the United Kingdom, the senior leaders and directors of OIRs at community colleges, and the heads of various professional associations who participated in the study and provided thoughtful comments and advice on how to establish a research and evaluation capability in METC. We are equally grateful to the VHA senior leaders who took time out of their busy schedules to talk with us about their organization's efforts to transform itself into a high-performing organization.

Several current and former RAND colleagues contributed to the study. We owe an enormous debt of gratitude to our reviewers, Catherine Augustine and Catherine Jackson, who gave us excellent suggestions for improving the clarity, flow, and readability of this monograph. We also thank former RAND colleagues, Marisa Adelson and Amber Price for their invaluable research assistance and enthusiasm. We particularly thank former RAND colleague Heather Barney for her excellent review and summary of several key components of the study during its early phases. RAND colleagues Amanda Scoggins and Hans Pung conducted the research on DMETA. Beth Asch, Susan Hosek, and Terri Tanielian provided useful comments as the study progressed and reviewed earlier drafts of the monograph. Finally, we thank Lauren Skrabala for her careful and patient editing and for putting up with us, yet again.

Abbreviations

ABHES	Accrediting Bureau of Health Education Schools
AIR	Association for Institutional Research
BRAC	Base Realignment and Closure
COE	Council on Occupational Education
CRCC	Community College Research Center
DMETA	Defence Medical Education and Training Agency
DoD	U.S. Department of Defense
DSAT	Defence Systems Approach to Training
ExVal	external validation
GAO	U.S. Government Accountability Office (formerly, U.S. General Accounting Office)
InVal	internal validation
IR	institutional research
MBNQA	Malcolm Baldrige National Quality Award
METC	medical education and training campus
MHS	Military Health System
MoD	UK Ministry of Defence

NCOD	National Center for Organizational Development
NDRI	RAND National Defense Research Institute
OIR	office of institutional research
ROI	return on investment
SACS	Southern Association of Colleges and Schools
VA	U.S. Department of Veterans Affairs
VHA	Veterans Health Administration
VISN	Veterans Integrated Service Network

CHAPTER ONE

Introduction

Over the past few years, there has been increasing recognition that the Military Health System (MHS) has to transform itself and the way it does business, given the changing environment: the rapid escalation in the costs of health care, the unprecedented challenges facing the military at home and abroad that require new roles and responsibilities, and the need to transform the medical force so that future medical support is fully aligned with joint force concepts. The 2005 Base Realignment and Closure (BRAC) Commission and the 2006 Quadrennial Defense Review provided more recent impetus and specific guidance for MHS transformation. In particular, the BRAC report recommended relocating basic and specialty enlisted medical training to Fort Sam Houston, Texas, to take advantage of economies of scale and facilitate the opportunity for joint training. To fulfill the BRAC recommendation, a joint medical education and training campus (METC) is being established at Fort Sam Houston. As of 2010, the plan is to colocate the three service schools and to consolidate medical training for all services to the extent feasible. The transition to METC is being overseen and guided by a jointly staffed executive integrated process team, under the guidance of a flag officer steering committee and a senior advisory council comprising the surgeons general of the Army, Navy, and Air Force. The vision is for METC to become the nation's leading military medical education and training institution, and its stated goals are to capture best practices and achieve efficiencies in training, i.e., to transform itself into a high-performing "learning" organization.

RAND was asked to provide technical and research assistance to METC in several areas related to (1) joint and service-specific scope of practice for enlisted medical specialties to foster interoperability of medical personnel, (2) joint leader development to ensure that military health care leaders are prepared to perform successfully in joint and performance-based environments, and (3) the need for and feasibility of establishing a research and evaluation capability within METC. This monograph documents the results of this third task; companion publications (Thie et al., 2009; Kirby and Thie, 2009; and Kirby et al., 2010) document RAND research and analysis related to the first two tasks.

Before we discuss the specifics of this monograph, we provide a brief overview of METC to set the context.

Overview of the Joint Medical Education and Training Campus

METC is a large, integrated campus under a single university-like administration; it officially opened its doors on June 30, 2010. Billed as the world's largest military medical training institution, it will be responsible for more than 100 enlisted medical training courses. METC began training personnel in April 2010, with its first course, Radiography Specialist. Other basic and specialty enlisted medical courses will be phased in over several months, with full operational capability expected in October 2011.

The courses are designed primarily for new soldiers, sailors, and airmen as part of their initial entry training. These courses will lead to award of an Army military occupational specialty, Air Force Specialty Code, or a Navy rating or Navy enlisted classification. Some students will return after one or more operational assignments for more-advanced training.

When fully operational, METC will have a yearly throughput of close to 25,000 students, an average daily student load of about 8,000, and an operating staff and faculty of more than 1,400. The courses offered will range from patient administration (the shortest course, at four weeks) to cytology (one of the longest, at 52 weeks). Most of the courses consist of two phases: a preliminary didactic phase and a clinical phase. For example, the cytology course is split into two approximately equal phases. The clinical phase may be conducted at medical facilities in the San Antonio area or elsewhere. Some courses have few students, while others, such as the Army's Health Care Specialist, will have an average student load of about 2,500.

Each service has its own entry requirements for these specialties. For the basic courses, these requirements typically include a high school diploma, mathematics or science courses, and minimum scores on the Armed Service Vocational Aptitude Battery. For the specialist or more-advanced courses, they include minimum operational time, grade requirements, educational prerequisites, and minimum time remaining in service. Currently, each service trains most of its specialists differently because of differences in standards of practice or military operational environments. METC's charge is to exploit economies of scale by offering consolidated training across the three services to the extent feasible. This will help promote interoperability across the services, another important driver of the BRAC recommendation to colocate the service schools. A key player in this work is the Health Care Interservice Training Office, which reviews service training curricula for the medical specialties, looking for commonalities with a view to recommending consolidated training, where feasible.

When fully operational, METC will offer more than 100 enlisted medical training courses in 38 academic programs:

- Advanced Dental Assistant
- Advanced Dental Laboratory
- Allergy/Immunology
- Animal Care Specialist
- Armed Forces Basic Medical Technician
- Basic Dental Laboratory
- Behavioral Health Technician
- Cardiopulmonary Lab Apprentice
- Cardiovascular Technology
- Cytotechnology
- Dental Assistant
- Department of Defense Biomedical Equipment Technician
- Electroneurodiagnostic Technician
- Health Physics Specialty
- Health Systems Management
- Hemodialysis/Apheresis

- Histopathology
- Independent Duty Medicine Technician
- Medical Laboratory
- Medical Logistics
- Nuclear Medical Technician
- Nutrition and Diet Therapy
- Occupational Therapy Assistant
- Ophthalmic Technician
- Optician
- Orthopedic
- Otolaryngology Technologist

- Patient Administration Specialist
- Pharmacy Technician
- Physical Therapist Assistant
- Practical Nurse
- Preventive Dentistry
- Preventive Medicine
- Radiography Specialist
- Respiratory Therapy Technician
- Surgical Technologist
- Urology Technician
- Veterinary Food Inspection Specialist.

Research Questions, Approach, and Organization of This Monograph

Our study addressed two major research questions:

1. Does METC need a research and evaluation capability?
2. What lessons can be learned from institutions with missions similar to that of METC in terms of research and evaluation activities and the structure and scope of an office of institutional research (OIR)?

We discuss each of these issues in turn, providing an overview of the approach and data used to answer each question.

Does METC Need a Research and Evaluation Capability?

To answer the first question, we undertook two research tasks. First, we used as a starting point METC's avowed goal of becoming a high-performing organization and examined the relevant literature to determine the role that research and evaluation play in such institutions. Senge (1990a, p. 3) defines learning organizations as organizations where people continually expand their capacity to create the results they truly desire, where new and expansive patterns of thinking are nurtured, where collective aspiration is set free, and where people are continually learning how to learn together.

Such organizations generally implement models of organizational improvement that allow them to collect, organize, and use data in a continuous-feedback loop designed to maximize the effectiveness of the learning process. We examined several models of organizational improvement. Because these models share several common features, we selected one—the framework used by the Malcolm Baldrige National Quality Award (MBNQA) program, established by Public Law 100-107 in 1987 as the U.S. national quality program—to highlight in this monograph. MBQNA establishes criteria for performance excellence and, in particular, has been adapted for the education sector. We also highlight one community college that was a 2005 MBQNA award winner.

Second, we focused on accreditation requirements. This focus grew out of discussions that METC might one day seek accreditation as a separate college rather than being accredited under another's accreditation umbrella. We examined the websites of three accreditation organizations that may be the most appropriate for METC: the Southern Association of Colleges and Schools (SACS), which is the regional accrediting body for degree-granting institutions in Texas; the Council on Occupational Education (COE), which is a national accrediting body for non–degree-granting and applied associate's degree–granting postsecondary occupational education institutions and has, in the past, accredited a variety of military training institutions; and the Accrediting Bureau of Health Education Schools (ABHES), which is a national accrediting body for degree and non–degree-granting institutions specializing in allied health. We focused particularly on requirements linked to research and evaluation. Accreditation bodies are increasingly requiring programs and institutions to develop and implement quality-improvement plans and learning objectives and to provide credible evidence of the value added to student learning and subsequent workforce outcomes.

The results of these two tasks are documented in Chapters Two and Three.

What Lessons Can Be Learned from Institutions with Similar Missions?

To answer the second question and to determine the role that research and evaluation play within institutions with missions similar to that of METC, as well as where this responsibility devolves, we undertook three research tasks.

First, because METC is similar to a community college offering technical training and eventually hopes to become an accredited community college, we conducted a series of interviews with the heads of OIRs at selected colleges (both community colleges and four-year undergraduate institutions) that matched METC in terms of student enrollment or that were widely regarded as exemplars. We also asked respondents about professional associations and networks with which typical OIRs are affiliated and interviewed representatives of these organizations. More details are provided in Chapter Four.

Second, recognizing that METC's mission is more limited than that of a traditional college (in the sense that it will offer primarily technical training rather than more general education), we looked to institutions that were more akin to METC in terms of focus on training. These included corporate universities; the Defence Medical Education and Training Agency (DMETA) in the United Kingdom, which closely mirrors METC in its mission and focus; and other federal agencies that emphasize the training and development of their staff.

METC resembles a corporate university, defined by Allen (2002, p. 9) as "an educational entity that is a strategic tool designed to assist its parent organization in achieving its mission by conducting activities that foster individual and organizational learning, knowledge and wisdom." Corporate universities offer a range of training to new employees and incumbent workers to ensure that they remain updated and current in the knowledge and skills needed to do their jobs. For example, they often offer technical skill training and job skill training to new employees and soft skill training (e.g., customer service, communication, problem solving, planning, project management), technical skill training, and job skill training to incumbent employees (Bober and Bartlett, 2004). METC is a "corporate" university designed to provide specific training in support of the mission of the MHS. As a result, we drew on existing literature to determine the types of research and evaluation—typically, evaluation of training programs—conducted by corporate universities.

As part of the larger project, we conducted a case study of DMETA, which was established by the UK Ministry of Defence (MoD) in 2003 to provide joint education and training for military medical personnel in the three services (British Army, Royal Navy, and Royal Air Force). It comes under the Joint Medical Command, a joint service agency whose mission is to provide secondary-care personnel to meet requirements for operational deployments and to support frontline units by educating and training medical personnel. We conducted two sets of interviews with senior staff at DMETA headquarters at Fort Blockhouse, Gosport, in 2007. We reviewed DMETA's website and documents provided to us by DMETA staff. The focus was on DMETA's structure and governance and how it designed and conducted joint training for the services. As part of our study, we reviewed DMETA's research and evaluation activities to see whether they might offer useful lessons for METC.

As part of a review of how federal agencies were addressing their human capital challenges, the U.S. Government Accountability Office (GAO) reviewed training and development efforts in selected federal agencies, including the Veterans Health Administration (VHA), to distill lessons learned and best practices. We reviewed these reports, focusing on research and evaluation activities. In addition, as part of the larger project, we conducted a case study of the VHA, focusing on its approach to leader development, interviewing several senior leaders, and reviewing documents provided to us. We selected the VHA for two reasons: (1) it is similar in size and mission to the U.S. Department of Defense (DoD) and falls under a cabinet-level official, and (2) like DoD, it has made a serious commitment to strategic human capital development (see Kirby et al., 2010). The VHA offers a range of training programs for employees at all levels, from entry-level staff to senior leaders in executive positions. For example, the School at Work engages students in an eight-month program designed to help them climb the ladder from an entry-level health care employee to more advanced positions. Students attend classes for two hours a week to brush up on basic skills and develop individual career and learning plans. It is not the programs, per se, that were important for the purposes of this study, but the VHA's approach to evaluation and commitment to becoming a learning organization dedicated to the education and development of all its employees. In this monograph, we reprise the VHA's efforts to transform itself into a high-performing learning organization, its establishment of a central office to monitor organizational health, and its ongoing emphasis on evaluation in all its training efforts.

Third, because evaluation of training programs is a major focus of organizations with missions similar to that of METC, we reviewed the strategic framework outlined by the GAO. A few years ago, as part of its ongoing review of how government agencies were addressing their human capital challenges, the GAO outlined "a framework to serve as a flexible and useful guide in assessing how agencies plan, design, implement, and evaluate effective training and development programs that contribute to improved organizational performance and enhanced employee skills and competencies" (GAO, 2004c, p. i). In this monograph, we focus largely on the last component of the training and development process—evaluation—and discuss the GAO's recommendations for designing effective training evaluations.

The results of these tasks are documented in Chapters Four and Five. Chapter Four presents data and findings from our interviews with OIR directors, along with their recommendations regarding the structure and scope of a METC OIR. Chapter Five expands further on specific research and evaluation activities undertaken by corporate universities, DMETA, and the VHA that may be relevant to METC's mission and reviews guidelines offered by the GAO regarding best practices in the evaluation of training programs.

A final chapter, Chapter Six, summarizes our conclusions and recommendations. The monograph concludes with an appendix that presents the criteria and framework for the MBNQA program.

As a final note, while each of the services currently evaluates its medical training programs, most of these efforts are fairly limited in nature and scope. In any case, given the potential consolidation of courses at METC, the focus and nature of these evaluations might be affected. It is also not clear to what extent those responsible for the service evaluations will migrate to METC in terms of staffing. In our study, we did not make assumptions about the migration of research and evaluation capabilities from the services to METC. Instead, we simply outline a case for building a research and evaluation capability housed within an OIR or similar office from the inception. If experienced staff are assigned to METC, it will be easier to establish this kind of capability.

CHAPTER TWO

Need for a Research and Evaluation Capability: Becoming a High-Performing Organization

Public accountability, organizational improvement, and transformation into a high-performing organization have become major concerns of both public and private organizations, including educational institutions at all levels. Understanding the characteristics of high-performing organizations will help guide METC in its efforts to create institutional conditions that are conducive to continuous organizational learning and improvement.

Characteristics of High-Performing Organizations

In February 2004, the GAO convened a forum on high-performing organizations that brought together leaders and experts from the public, not-for-profit, and for-profit sectors as well as from academia and professional associations. As described in the subsequent report on the proceedings of the forum (GAO, 2004b), the purpose was to help the federal government build high-performing organizations that can meet the challenges of the 21st century:

> As we face the mounting challenges of the 21st century, the federal government must strive to build high-performing organizations. Nothing less than a fundamental transformation in the people, processes, technology, and environment used by federal agencies to address public goals will be necessary to address the public needs facing the nation in a time of rapid change. In high-performing organizations, management controls, processes, practices, and sys-

tems are adopted in areas such as financial management, information technology, acquisition management, and human capital that are consistent with prevailing best practices and that contribute to concrete organizational results. Ultimately, however, to successfully transform, the federal government needs to change its culture to become more results-oriented, client- and customer-focused, and collaborative in nature. (GAO, 2004b, p. 1)

Forum participants emphasized that high-performing organizations are focused on achieving results and outcomes and that, "to sustain a focus on results, high-performing organizations continuously assess and benchmark performance and efforts to improve performance" (GAO, 2004b, p. 7). Participants also identified key characteristics of high-performing organizations that supported this results-oriented focus. These included the following (GAO, 2004b, pp. 3–4):

- *A clear, well-articulated, and compelling mission.* High-performing organizations have a clear, well-articulated, and compelling mission; the strategic goals to achieve it; and a performance management system that aligns with these goals to show employees how their performance can contribute to overall organizational results. With these elements in place, regularly communicating a clear and consistent message about the importance of fulfilling the mission helps engage employees, clients, customers, partners, and other stakeholders in achieving higher performance.
- *Strategic use of partnerships.* This point is emphasized by all high-performing organizations. In particular, participants noted that, since the federal government is increasingly reliant on partners to achieve its outcomes, becoming a high-performing organization requires that federal agencies effectively manage relationships with other organizations outside their direct control.
- *Focus on needs of clients and customers.* Serving the needs of clients and customers involves identifying needs, striving to meet them, measuring performance, and publicly reporting on progress to help ensure appropriate transparency and accountability.
- *Strategic management of people.* Most high-performing organizations have strong, charismatic, visionary, and sustained leader-

ship; the capability to identify the skills and competencies that employees and the organization need; and other key characteristics, including effective recruiting, comprehensive training and development, retention of high-performing employees, and a streamlined hiring process.

At the heart of most high-performing organizations is an organizational improvement model or methodology—such as Total Quality Management, Lean Production, Six Sigma, and MBQNA, to name some of the more enduring models—that allows the organization to manage its business processes in an integrated way to further its goals. Implicit in all organizational improvement methodologies is the notion that, with attention to data and other signals, organizations can learn from their own behavior. Peter Senge (1990a) is often credited with popularizing the idea of the "learning organization," although subsequent researchers have added considerably to the theory of organizational change and learning. Lipshitz, Popper, and Friedman (2002, p. 82, quoting Barnett, undated, p. 9) define organizational learning as "an experience-based process through which knowledge about action-outcome relationships develops, is encoded in routines, is embedded in organizational memory, and changes collective behavior."

Implicit in this definition is the information-as-signal hypothesis, which suggests that when information about action-outcome relationships is available, organizations will respond to that information in positive ways to improve their performance (Huber, 1990). Thus, collecting, retrieving, analyzing, and learning from information can help organizations read their environment and adapt to change. Advocates of the learning organization paradigm view it as key to achieving a sustainable competitive advantage and necessary for organizational survival (De Gues, 1988; Drucker, 1999; Nonaka, 1991; Schein, 1993; Senge, 1990a, 1990b). The federal government has recognized the need to work better by improving efficiency and effectiveness. David Walker, U.S. Comptroller General from 1998 to 2008, reinforced the theme by stating that this goal requires government audit organizations to become learning organizations. They must be adept at understanding the purpose and objectives of government programs, the criteria for measuring their success, the research and analytical tools necessary to perform that measurement, and the skills and knowledge needed to fashion constructive solutions and recommendations to make those programs work better. (Walker, 2002)

More recently, Garvin, Edmondson, and Gino (2008, p. 109) pointed out that leaders often erroneously think that "getting their organizations to learn is *only* a matter of articulating a clear vision, giving employees the right incentives, and providing lots of training." They identified three factors that have impeded organizations' progress in attempting to transform into learning organizations:

First, many of the early discussions about learning organizations were paeans to a better world rather than concrete prescriptions. They overemphasized the forest and paid little attention to the trees. As a result, the associated recommendations proved difficult to implement—managers could not identify the sequence of steps necessary for moving forward. Second, the concept was aimed at CEOs and senior executives rather than at managers of smaller departments and units where critical organizational work is done. Those managers had no way of assessing how their teams' learning was contributing to the organization as a whole. Third, standards and tools for assessment were lacking. Without these, companies could declare victory prematurely or claim progress without delving into the particulars or comparing themselves accurately with others. (Garvin, Edmondson, and Gino, 2008, p. 109)

The federal government has continued this learning and performance emphasis by stressing it as its first strategy for achieving high performance. For example, the budget of the U.S. government recommends using performance information to lead, learn, and improve outcomes:

Government operates more effectively when it focuses on outcomes, when leaders set clear and measurable goals, and when agencies use measurement to reinforce priorities, motivate action, and illuminate a path to improvement. (Office of Management and Budget, 2010, p. 73)

Still, the theory of organizational learning and the information-as-signal hypothesis is not without complexities. A number of studies in the field have focused on understanding why organizations often fail to use information to produce learning and improved outcomes. Several researchers have suggested that data and information tend to have low relative importance in organizational decisionmaking due to the highly politicized nature of most decisions. Instead, ideology and vested interests tend to take precedence (Markus, 1983; Dean and Sharfman, 1993; Ostrom, 1990; Simon, 1991; Weiss, 1983). Feldman and March (1981) suggested that the role of information is primarily symbolic: Organizations advance the collection of data to convey the illusory sense of rationality but do not use it as a basis for actual decisions. Serenko, Bontis, and Hardie (2007) suggest that the effectiveness of internal knowledge flows and knowledge sharing diminishes as the size of an organizational unit increases. They infer that this is due to increased complexity in the formal structure, weaker interpersonal relationships, and less effective communication.

Some researchers have focused on the types of decisions that tend to lend themselves to information use and organizational learning and have found that decisionmakers are most likely to use information in highly structured problem contexts—when problems are difficult to define, solutions are not well known, and the certainty of outcomes is low. In other contexts, they tend to rely on tacit, intuitive knowledge (Choo, 1998; Daft, 1998; Daft and Macintosh, 1981; Turban, McLean, and Wetherbe, 1996). Others have suggested that organizational learning has as much to do with the culture of the organization as with the structures and processes put into place. For example, Nonaka and von Krogh (2009) discuss the interaction between tacit and explicit knowledge, stating that additional research is needed to understand how leadership can motivate and enable individuals to contribute to organizational knowledge creation by transcending social practices.

To become an organization in which employees excel at creating, acquiring, and transferring knowledge, an institution needs a supportive learning environment, concrete learning processes and practices, and leaders who by their behavior reinforce learning. What is clear from the literature is that simply putting key elements in place will not drive improvement unless they are well integrated into the organizational culture and linked to well-articulated performance goals.

As stated earlier, there is a host of models of organizational improvement, and all begin with a focus on data and information as signal but seek to provide specific tools and build cultures to avoid the pitfalls of unstructured information use. Because these models are fairly similar, we focus here on the Baldrige model.[1] Our decision to focus on this framework was not based not on evaluative criteria that one particular model or quality-improvement process was more important than another. Instead, it was driven by two considerations. First, the Baldrige framework underpins the MBNQA, arguably the most prestigious award for organizational excellence in the United States. Second, it has been adapted for the education sector. As such, it seems to be a more useful framework for METC to consider as the basis for its transformative efforts.

---

[1]   We should note that there are several quality awards—for example, the Deming Prize in Japan, the European Quality Award, and the Australian Quality Award—each of which is based on a perceived model of total quality management. Although there are some differences among the quality awards, they provide a universal audit framework for evaluating management practices; quality of methods, techniques, and tools; deployment of quality plans; and results. Ghobadian and Woo (1996) provide an excellent comparison of the characteristics of these four major quality awards, pointing out, for example, that—unlike the other three—the Deming Prize is not based on an underlying framework linking concepts and practices to results. Thus, it does not assume causality but is more prescriptive in that it recommends a list of desirable quality-oriented best practices, such as quality circles and standardization. The MBNQA, European Quality Award, and Australian Quality Award are based on an underlying causal framework linking different constituents of quality management and are prescriptive in the sense that they expound a particular philosophy of good management. Ghobadian and Woo do not recommend particular methods or tools, however.

Malcolm Baldrige National Quality Award Program

The goal of the Malcolm Baldrige National Quality Act of 1987 (Public Law 100-107) is to establish criteria for performance excellence and to provide organizations with a framework for designing, implementing, and assessing a process for managing all business or organizational operations and meeting those criteria.[2] We provide some background on the MBNQA program and its criteria for performance excellence; a more detailed discussion is presented in the appendix. Kirby (2004) reviews the evidence regarding the link between implementation of the MBNQA framework and operating performance; we do not review that topic here. Instead, we discuss how these criteria have been applied to the education sector.

Background

Congress established the MBNQA program "to promote quality awareness, to recognize quality and business achievements of U.S. organizations, and to publicize these organizations' successful performance strategies" (NIST, 2009). The award recognizes performance excellence in each of the following five categories: manufacturing, service, small business, and (starting in 1999) education and health care. Up to three awards may be given in each category per year, although in some areas and some years, no awards are given if applicants are judged as not meeting the standards. The award is not given for a specific product or service but for meeting the criteria for performance excellence.[3]

---

[2] This section is largely drawn from Kirby (2004).

[3] The U.S. Commerce Department's National Institute of Standards and Technology manages the MBNQA program with assistance from the American Society for Quality, a professional nonprofit association. The award program is a joint public-private effort. Volunteers serve as members of the MBNQA Board of Examiners to review applications, make site visits, and make recommendations regarding awards. The board comprises more than 500 experts from industry, educational institutions, all levels of government, and nonprofit organizations who go through a training process to become Baldrige examiners. Organizations that wish to apply for an award must submit an eligibility determination package to establish eligibility in one of the five award categories. Once an organization is determined to be eligible, it submits a completed application form along with an application report consisting of an organizational overview and responses to the criteria for performance excellence.

The MBNQA performance excellence criteria provide a framework that any organization can use to improve overall performance. Seven categories make up the award criteria and are discussed in greater detail in the appendix:

- leadership
- strategic planning
- customer focus
- measurement, analysis, and knowledge management
- workforce focus
- process management
- results.

Education Criteria for Performance Excellence

In 1999, the MBNQA program was extended to the education and health sectors.[4] This expansion assumed that the same seven-part framework underlying the business criteria was adaptable to all organizations, but it also recognized that the guidelines needed some adaptation to fit these new sectors. The underlying belief was that using the same framework for all sectors of the economy would foster cross-sector learning and sharing of information on best practices. Any for-profit or not-for-profit public or private organization that provides educational services in the United States or its territories is eligible to apply for the award, including elementary and secondary schools and school districts; colleges, universities, and university systems; schools or col-

---

All applicants receive a detailed feedback report, a written assessment of the organization's strengths and vulnerabilities that contains detailed, actionable comments on opportunities for improvement. Several organizations have praised the quality and usefulness of the feedback (see NIST, 2009).

Another important emphasis of the program is dissemination. Recipients of the award are asked to participate in an annual conference at which the awards are announced, and several have cosponsored regional conferences. They are also expected to share basic materials on their organizations' performance strategies and methods and to answer news media inquiries.

[4]   This section draws heavily on the program's *2009–2010 Education Criteria for Performance Excellence* (Baldrige National Quality Program, 2009).

leges within a university; professional schools; community colleges; and technical schools.

The purpose of the education criteria is to provide organizations with an integrated approach to organizational performance management that will help them deliver ever-improving value to students and stakeholders, contributing to education quality and organizational stability, improving overall organizational effectiveness and capabilities, and fostering organizational and personal learning. The criteria are built on a set of interrelated core values and concepts that are embedded in systematic processes yielding performance results. The Baldrige program posits that these values and concepts

> are embedded beliefs and behaviors found in high-performing organizations. They are the foundation for integrating key performance and operational requirements within a results-oriented framework that creates a basis for action and feedback. (Baldrige National Quality Program, 2009, p. 51)

These core values and concepts, which are described in this monograph's appendix, include the following:

- visionary leadership
- learning-centered education
- organizational and personal learning
- valuing workforce members and partners
- agility
- focus on the future
- managing for innovation
- management by fact
- societal responsibility
- focus on results and creating value
- systems perspective.

As mentioned earlier, the Baldrige model of organizational improvement rests on a seven-part framework discussed in the appendix. Within each category, a number of questions help guide an organization's efforts to use the model for self-assessment or as a first step toward application. The framework emphasizes the role of measurement, analysis, and knowledge management, calling it the "brain center" for aligning the organization's programs and offerings with its strategic objectives. Organizations are asked to consider how they select and use data for performance measurement, analysis, and review to support organizational planning and performance improvement and how they ensure that the data collected are relevant for decisionmaking.

Award Winners

Since the inception of the Education category, eight educational institutions have won the Baldrige award (see text box).[5]

Richland Community College is the first and only community college to receive the MBNQA in education.[6] It serves a multicultural student body of about 14,500 students seeking college credit and about 6,000 continuing education students. In setting and deploying its vision and values, direction, and performance expectations, it sought input from a broad range of stakeholders, including students, faculty, staff, and community members. It identified four strategic planning priorities: identify and meet community educational needs, enable all students to succeed, enable all employees to succeed, and ensure institutional effectiveness, each with its own measures for success, called "key performance indicators." Systematic data collection ensures that information is readily available to support fact-based decisionmaking, helping the college remain agile and innovative. Its senior leadership team, the "ThunderTeam," meets monthly to review these indicators and the progress being made in meeting the four priorities. If progress seems to be lagging, the ThunderTeam asks its members to "drill down" into the organization for root causes and to suggest actions to improve performance. Richland participates in several networks aimed at organizational improvement, including the League for Innovation

---

[5] The program posts profiles, application summaries, and contact information for all its award winners on its website as part of its dissemination process.

[6] Information about Richland College is drawn from its profile and award application summary available at Baldrige National Quality Program (2005) and Richland College (2005), respectively.

Winners of the Malcolm Baldrige National Quality Award in Education, 1999–2009

2001:

Chugach School District, a preschool through postsecondary school system in South Central Alaska, serving 214 students spread across 22,000 square miles

Pearl River School District, a K–12 public school system in Rockland County, New York, serving 2,500 students and offering continuing education to 1,000 adults

University of Wisconsin-Stout, one of 13 publicly supported universities in the University of Wisconsin system in Menomonie, Wisconsin, serving 8,000 students and offering both undergraduate and graduate programs

2003:

Community Consolidated School District 15, a K–8 public school system in Palatine, Illinois (a northwestern Chicago suburb), serving approximately 12,500 students, many of whom come from low-income and non–English-speaking families

2004:

Kenneth W. Montfort College of Business, a college within the University of Northern Colorado in Greeley, Colorado, graduating about 300 students per year

2005:

Jenks Public Schools, a pre-K–12 school district serving about 10,000 students located just south of Tulsa, Oklahoma, and the 11th largest school district in Oklahoma

Richland Community College, one of seven two-year community colleges in the Dallas Community College District, serving about 14,500 students seeking college credit and 6,000 continuing education students

2008:

Iredell-Statesville Schools, a K–12 public school system in southwestern North Carolina, serving about 21,000 students

SOURCE: Baldrige National Quality Program, 2010b.

NOTE: There were no award recipients in the education category in the years not shown.

---

in the Community College and the Continuous Quality Improvement Network. Benchmarking against peers and competitors is an important component of its performance improvement strategy. In addition to the MBQNA, Richland has won a number of awards, including the Texas Award for Performance Excellence in 2005, and has been recognized by several other organizations (for example, the American Association of Colleges and Universities named Richland one of 16 institutions noted for visionary campus-wide innovation in undergraduate education).

While there is no hard evidence linking the adoption of and feedback from the Baldrige improvement process to improved performance, testimonials from the winners of the award suggest that they believe that the two are related. Most point to increased enrollment, increased retention, and increased graduation rates, as well as improved performance by students on various achievement tests. Some also cite decreased turnover among staff. Richland, for example, highlighted (1) a threefold increase in the number of students who completed the core curriculum in preparation for transfer to four-year institutions from 2002 to 2005, (2) student satisfaction measures that are higher than national norms, (3) a higher-than-average (among peers) increase in enrollment among credit students, and (4) the career success of several former employees who became presidents of other colleges.

It is clear that such testimonials do not provide evidence of cause and effect. Nonetheless, the process, the feedback, and being part of a network of like-minded organizations may prove salutary. As the Baldrige website claims:

> Baldrige applicants know that the journey is not about receiving a Presidential Award, although that's a nice goal. It's about getting expert feedback on where they are and where they need to be. It's about having the tools to examine all parts of their management model and improve processes while keeping the whole organization in mind. (Baldrige National Quality Program, 2010a)

Implications for METC

The education criteria provide guidelines on conducting an institutional self-assessment based on a detailed organizational profile and developing a strategic plan linked to clearly identified goals and reinforced by an information and analysis system to collect data and monitor progress toward those goals. In addition, the education criteria are designed to help educational institutions use an integrated approach to organizational performance management with a view to enhancing overall organizational effectiveness and capabilities and improving learning among students, faculty, and the organization itself. Developing a detailed organizational profile is the first step in the Baldrige process. The discipline imposed by having to clearly articulate the environment in which the organization operates, the organization's culture (purpose, mission, vision, and goals), its structure and governance system, its key stakeholders, the regulatory environment, key partner relationships, and the major technologies, equipment, and facilities available could be very useful to METC.

For our purposes, regardless of which improvement model METC adopts, it is clear that measurement, analysis, and knowledge management serve as the foundation for the performance management system and are critical to a fact-based, knowledge-driven system for improving performance. Thus, to support its goal of becoming a high-performing organization, METC will need to develop and sustain the capability to collect, organize, analyze, and use data on a variety of processes and outcomes to support innovation and performance excellence. In addition, it will need to review these indicators and data and analysis systems on a periodic basis to adapt to new or changing environments and stakcholder needs.

CHAPTER THREE

Need for a Research and Evaluation Capability: Accreditation Requirements

When METC is fully established, it will be responsible for training personnel in more than 100 enlisted medical specialties and will be the world's largest military medical education and training institution, with an average daily student load of more than 8,000 and a total of 1,400 faculty and staff members. Many of the programs require program accreditation. In the case of the Air Force, enlisted service members can obtain academic credit for the courses they attend. To be able to grant such credit, METC plans to affiliate with the Community College of the Air Force, which is accredited by SACS through the Air University.[1] Early on in planning, it was discussed that METC may one day seek formal accreditation as a degree-granting institution of higher education, accessible to members of all the services.

Accreditation in higher education requires an external quality review by a private, nonprofit organization. In the United States, accreditation is the primary "stamp of approval" indicating that an institution provides a legitimate education that meets standards of quality. Accreditation is often a requirement for eligibility for state and federal grants and loans. In addition, students are required to attend an accredited institution in order to receive certain types of federal and state financial aid and to sit for licensure examinations in some professions.

---

[1] The Community College of the Air Force was separately accredited by SACS from 1980 to 2004. Since 2004, it shares the Air University's regional accreditation (see Air University, undated).

In the United States, 19 organizations accredit higher-education institutions. Six regional organizations accredit within specific geographic areas and tend to accredit only degree-granting, nonprofit institutions. In addition, 13 national organizations accredit entire institutions without regard to location.[2] Table 3.1 lists accrediting organizations with missions relevant to METC's program.

Individual programs within an institution may also be accredited. As with institutional accreditation, programmatic accreditation serves as an indicator that an educational program has met specific standards for quality.

The following sections review accreditation processes and standards in three institutional accreditation organizations that may be most appropriate for METC: SACS, the regional accrediting body for degree-granting institutions in Texas; COE, a national accrediting body for non–degree-granting and applied associate's degree–granting postsecondary occupational education institutions and has in the past accredited a variety of military training institutions; and ABHES, a

Table 3.1
Selected Institutional Accreditation Organizations

Regional	Private National
Middle States Association of Colleges and Schools	Accrediting Bureau of Health Education Schools
New England Association of Schools and Colleges	Accrediting Commission of Career Schools and Colleges
North Central Association of Colleges and Schools	Accrediting Council for Continuing Education and Training
Northwest Commission on Colleges and Universities	Council on Occupational Education
Southern Association of Colleges and Schools	Distance Education and Training Council
Western Association of Schools and Colleges	

---

[2] Information about the general accreditation process and the accrediting organizations is from the Council on Higher Education Accreditation (undated).

national accrediting body for degree and non–degree-granting institutions specializing in allied health. Here, we focus primarily on the requirements that may present substantive issues for METC.

Southern Association of Colleges and Schools

SACS is the regional accrediting body for degree-granting institutions in Virginia, North Carolina, South Carolina, Georgia, Florida, Alabama, Mississippi, Tennessee, Kentucky, Louisiana, and Texas.[3] Its Commission on Colleges accredits all institutions granting associate's, bachelor's, master's, and doctoral degrees. Both the Air University at Maxwell Air Force Base in Alabama and the Marine Corps University in Quantico, Virginia, are accredited through SACS (see SACS, 2010). About one-third of its members are associate's degree–granting institutions.

The SACS Commission on Colleges bases its accreditation on requirements in the *Principles of Accreditation: Foundations for Quality Enhancement.* These principles apply to all applicant, candidate, and member institutions, regardless of the type of institution (private for-profit, private not-for-profit, or public). The commission evaluates an institution and makes accreditation decisions based on compliance with its principle of integrity (Section 1), core requirements (Section 2), comprehensive standards (Section 3), additional federal requirements (Section 4), and other policies.

Institutions interested in learning more about or seeking accreditation must first attend a one-day workshop at the commission's offices. The purpose of the workshop is to acquaint attendees with the accreditation process and requirements. The initial application requires documentation of compliance with the following criteria:

---

[3]   All information about SACS is from the website of its Commission on Colleges (SACS, undated), the 2010 version of its *Principles of Accreditation* (SACS, 2009a), its *Resource Manual for the Principles of Accreditation* (SACS, 2005), and its *Handbook for Institutions Seeking Reaffirmation* (SACS, 2009b).

- 11 out of 12 core requirements relating to (among others) degree-granting authority, roles and responsibilities of the governing board and chief executive officer, institutional mission, institutional effectiveness, program length and content, faculty qualifications, and student support services
- three out of 14 comprehensive standards relating to institutional effectiveness, college-level competencies, and faculty qualifications
- federal regulations relating to (among others) student achievement, program curriculum, publication of policies, student complaints as specified under Title IV of the 1998 Higher Education Amendments (Public Law 105-244).

Once the application has been reviewed, a candidacy committee makes a site visit to the institution to verify the documentation and submits a report to the Committee on Compliance and Reports, which recommends the institution for candidacy status. Once an institution has been accepted as a candidate, it must document compliance with the additional comprehensive standards and receive a site visit from an accreditation committee within two years. The accreditation committee makes a recommendation for membership, continued candidacy (in which case the institution has two more years to document compliance), or removal of candidacy. Member institutions must have their accreditation reaffirmed after five years, which requires documentation and verification of compliance with all standards and requirements from the initial accreditation as well as the 12th core requirement, which concerns the institution's quality-enhancement plan.

Council on Occupational Education

COE is a national organization that accredits non–degree-granting and associate's degree–granting career and technical schools, including several military training institutions.[4]

---

[4] All information about COE is from its website (COE, undated) and the 2010 edition of its *Handbook of Accreditation* (COE, 2010).

Institutions begin the accreditation process by submitting an application for candidacy. Following receipt of the application, COE sends a two-person team to conduct a two-day site visit. The council's Commission on Occupational Education Institutions reviews the institution's application and financial statements, as well as the report of the site-visit team and the institutional response, and votes on the candidacy application. Once a candidate, an institution sends a representative to a self-study workshop and completes an institutional self-study. At least six months after the workshop (but not more than 18 months later), the institution hosts a four-day accreditation team visit. The team leader makes a preliminary visit one month prior to the full team visit, at which point the self-study must be complete. The accreditation team writes a site-visit report, and the institution has 30 days to respond in writing to any specific recommendations. The commission reviews the self-study, the site-visit report, and the institutional response and determines whether or not to grant accreditation.

Renewal of accreditation status requires submission of an annual report to COE. Reaffirmation occurs once every two to six years and requires attendance at the self-study workshop, completion of an institutional self-study, and an accreditation team site visit.

COE accreditation standards relate to (among others) institutional mission, educational programs, program and institutional outcomes, strategic planning, and learning and support resources for students. All standards must be met for accreditation and reaffirmation. In addition, selected documentation related to the standards is required for candidacy.

Accrediting Bureau of Health Education Schools

ABHES is a national accrediting body for degree and non–degree-granting institutions specializing in allied health.[5]

---

[5] All information about ABHES is from the organization's website (ABHES, undated) and the 16th edition of its *Accreditation Manual* (ABHES, 2010).

Institutions begin the accreditation process by submitting an application for accreditation. Once ABHES has accepted the application, a representative conducts a preliminary visit to provide additional information on the accreditation process and to assess the degree to which the institution's current practices meet the accreditation standards. If the report from this preliminary visit is satisfactory, the institution submits a self-evaluation report. ABHES requires that all initial and renewal applicants seeking accreditation attend an accreditation workshop prior to submission of the completed self-evaluation report. A visitation team that generally includes at least one academic and one administrator conducts a site visit and writes a visitation team report, to which the institution has three weeks to respond. After a full review by the bureau's Preliminary Review Committee, the ABHES Board of Commissioners considers all relevant documentation and determines whether or not to accredit the institution. Standards cover such topics as mission and objectives, administration and management, programs, and satisfactory academic outcomes. In addition, institutions that offer occupational and applied science or academic associate's degrees must meet a set of degree program standards relating to (among others) faculty qualifications, learning resources, student services, and curriculum.

Substantive Issues of Relevance to METC

The majority of the standards and requirements for all three accrediting bodies are relatively generic and nonprescriptive. For example, they require that the institution have control over particular programs or that a policy for a given topic exists and is published and enforced, but they do not specify any requirements for the content of the program. Other standards require that a given service or program be "adequate" or "appropriate" to the institution's mission but do not define these terms or specify particular requirements. A few of the standards and requirements do, however, present substantive specifications that should be considered if accreditation is a long-term goal for METC.

Degree-Granting Authority

To be accredited, institutions must have degree-granting authority from the appropriate government agency. In METC's case, this may require approval from Congress.

Institutional Independence

With specific regard to military institutions, SACS requires that the presiding officer of the board and the majority of its members be neither civilian employees of the military nor active or retired military. In addition, the presiding officer and the majority of voting members must be free from contractual, employment, and financial interest in the institution. Similarly, COE requires the institution to have an advisory committee with the majority of the membership external to the institution. To meet the SACS specifications, the Air University and Marine Corps University established boards of visitors with majority civilian membership to advise their commanding officers.

Program Length

All three organizations specify that programs must require at least 60 credit hours for an associate's degree, of which at least 15 must be in general education. COE further defines one credit hour as the equivalent of 15 clock hours of lecture, 30 clock hours of lab work, or 45 clock hours of work-based learning. ABHES has additional requirements for specific degrees. For example, programs leading to an associate of applied science, associate of art, or associate of science degree must include at least 15 hours of general education and 30 hours in the occupational area of the degree, while those leading to an associate of occupational science degree must include nine hours of general education and 45 hours in the occupational area. For all degree programs, at least 25 percent of required credits must be completed at the institution.

Faculty Qualifications

SACS requires that faculty who teach courses at the associate's level for which credit will not be applied to a bachelor's program have a bachelor's degree in the teaching discipline or an associate's degree and demonstrated competency in the teaching discipline. Similarly, COE requires technical faculty in associate's degree programs to have at least an associate's degree. ABHES requires instructors of occupational courses to have graduated from an accredited program in the teaching specialty, a minimum of three years of job-related training and experience, and current licenses or certifications, as required for their occupational specialty. For academic associate's degree programs, at least 50 percent of courses offered must be taught by faculty with a bachelor's degree or higher, and at least 50 percent of general education courses must be taught by faculty with a master's degree or higher.

Program Evaluation, Assessment, and Improvement

All three accrediting bodies emphasize the importance of program evaluation, assessment, and improvement. For example, SACS requires that

> the institution engages in ongoing, integrated, and institution-wide research-based planning and evaluation processes that (1) incorporate a systematic review of institutional mission, goals, and outcomes; (2) result in continuing improvement in institutional quality; and (3) demonstrate that the institution is effectively accomplishing its mission. (SACS, 2009a, p. 16)

In addition, it requires that "the institution identifies expected outcomes, assesses the extent to which it achieves these outcomes, and provides evidence of improvement based on analysis of the results" (SACS, 2009a, p. 25). SACS expects outcomes to be defined and measured in the following areas: educational programs (including student learning outcomes), administrative and educational support services, and research and community or public service relevant to the institution's educational mission, as appropriate. It also suggests the use of periodic reviews of programmatic outcomes, such as graduation rates and employer and alumni satisfaction.

Similarly, COE lists several outcome indicators that institutions must track, including program completion data, program placement data, licensure exam performance, evaluation of knowledge and skills for the occupation, and information from employers regarding program effectiveness. Information on these indicators must be made available to all institutional personnel at least annually. It also requires that each educational program be reviewed at least every two years by a committee composed of at least three external employers in the program field. The institution must have a written strategic plan with objectives for at least a three-year time frame, strategies for plan evaluation, and annual reporting on results.

ABHES requires each accredited program to have a program effectiveness plan that

> establishes and documents specific goals, collects outcome data relevant to these goals, analyzes outcomes against both minimally acceptable benchmarks and the program's short- and long-term objectives, and sets strategies to improve program performance (ABHES, 2010, p. 62).

Program effectiveness is judged by program retention rates, job placement rates, credentialing examination participation and pass rates, and faculty participation in professional growth and in-service activities, as well as the program's participation in required surveys of students, graduates, clinical affiliates, and employers and their level of satisfaction with the program. Programs must also show that they measure and track outcomes and provide a summary and analysis of data collected for continuous improvement.

Implications for METC

This chapter reviewed the process and requirements for accreditation with three institutional accrediting bodies (SACS, COE, and ABHES) whose missions seem best aligned with METC's proposed purpose and structure. While standards for all three are relatively nonprescriptive, a handful of standards may present larger substantive issues for METC, particularly those related to governance structures, program length, and faculty credentials. Regardless of the accrediting body with which METC chooses to align itself, we note that institutional improvement and assessment are important factors in the standards of all of the institutional accrediting organizations in the United States.[6]

Nearly all higher-education accrediting organizations require institutions to produce some form of written improvement plan on a regular basis. Most have several common features. For example, plans typically must include measurable short- and longer-term (three to five years) objectives, as well as benchmarks, a plan and timeline for implementation, consideration of necessary resources, and a plan for evaluation with measurable outcomes. Plans are generally expected to include explicit links to the institution's mission and goals. In most cases, the accreditation standards call for broad-based participation from all or many institutional stakeholders and constituencies. Several organizations also require consideration of the institutional context, which may include such mitigating factors as the characteristics of the student body or the state of the local labor market. Finally, all standards related to written improvement plans include requirements that the progress of implementation of the plans be evaluated and assessed, typically on an annual basis.

Several organizations specifically define the cyclical nature of evaluation processes; for example, the Middle States Association of Colleges and Schools standards describe a four-step planning and assessment cycle that includes defining goals, implementing strategies, assessing achievement of the goals, and using assessment results to inform and improve programs and services. It and several other organizations also call for assessment and evaluation to be a part of all aspects of the institution, including not only educational programs but also student

---

[6] We reviewed the websites of several other accrediting bodies, including the Accrediting Commission for Career Schools and Colleges of Technology, the Accrediting Council for Continuing Education and Training, the Accrediting Council for Independent Colleges and Schools, the Middle States Association of Colleges and Schools, the North Central Association of Schools and Colleges, the Western Association of Schools and Colleges, the New England Association of Schools and Colleges, the Northwest Commission on Colleges and Universities, and the Distance Education and Training Council.

services, human resources, library and information resources, physical facilities, and so on. In addition, the effectiveness of the assessment and evaluation processes themselves should be systematically reviewed.

The standards of the various accrediting organizations also specify a range of quality indicators that may be used for assessment and evaluation of occupational education programs, including

- graduation or completion rate
- employment or placement rate
- pass rate on professional licensure exams
- employer satisfaction
- participant satisfaction
- retention
- attendance
- student progress
- assessment of occupational skills and knowledge.

Notably, several of these indicators (licensure exam pass rate, employer satisfaction, placement rate) require follow-up with program graduates. In addition, several organizations provide benchmarks for certain indicators (such as graduation rates or licensure exam pass rates), typically determined by evaluating data from current organizational members or peer institutions. For example, the Accrediting Commission for Career Schools and Colleges of Technology requires that institutions' graduation and employment rates not be less than one standard deviation below that of comparable schools or programs.

Should METC seek accreditation in the future, it will need a research and evaluation capability to meet the accreditation requirement for institutional improvement plans, embedded assessment, and tracking of a variety of indicators.

CHAPTER FOUR

Structure and Scope of an Office of Institutional Research: Findings from Interviews

This chapter examines the structure and scope of OIRs in two- and four-year postsecondary institutions. We draw on two data sources.

Data

The primary data source for this chapter is a series of interviews that we conducted with heads of OIRs at selected community colleges and four-year institutions, leaders in three professional associations (the Association for Institutional Research [AIR], the American Association of Community Colleges, and the League for Innovation in Community Colleges), and a representative of a major initiative, Achieving the Dream, which aims to transform community colleges. The sample of institutions was selected iteratively. We first selected three of the largest community college systems in the United States for our interviews because they might be more likely to adopt best practices that would be relevant for METC. In terms of enrollment, these institutions are considerably larger than METC's projected enrollment of 24,500 students. Our sample included Miami Dade College, Florida (170,000 students); Los Angeles Community College District, California (130,000 students); and Maricopa County Community College District, Arizona (250,000 students). In interviews with the heads of professional associations, we solicited advice about exemplars and information about other institutions that might offer lessons learned for METC with respect to the scope and governance of OIRs. This led to interviews with two smaller community colleges—South Texas

College (20,000 students) and Valencia Community College, Florida (50,000 students)—and four universities, including Tufts University, Massachusetts (9,500 students); University of Miami, Florida (15,000 students); Appalachian State University, North Carolina (16,500 students); and Indiana University (100,000 students).

We used a semistructured protocol for the interviews with the heads of the OIRs. Apart from the educational and career background of the respondent, we asked about the structure and governance of the OIR, its roles and functions (in particular, its role in the accreditation process and the institutional review board, which reviews research involving human subjects, as required by federal regulation),[1] and networks and professional associations in which the respondent participated as head of the OIR. We also solicited advice on establishing an OIR for METC. In interviewing leaders of professional organizations, we asked about the mission of the organization and services provided to educational institutions, especially to individuals involved in institutional research (IR) and planning. We also asked them to comment on the skills needed by those heading such offices and, more generally, for their advice for METC in setting up such an office. We also solicited recommendations regarding colleges and universities that might be useful to include in the study sample.

We analyzed the interview data and coded responses under broad categories: skills and education needed for OIR staff, governance and communication, scope and functions, examples of how reporting had influenced decisionmaking, networks and professional associations, and advice or recommendations for METC. We then looked for broad themes across the institutions and organizations, along with responses that seemed to be specific to certain types of institutions (for example, larger colleges or universities).

The second data source is a report published by the Community College Research Center (CRCC) at the Teachers College at Columbia University (Morest and Jenkins, 2007). As part of the Achieving the Dream initiative, CRCC conducted a study to see how well pre-

---

[1]   These requirements are outlined in the Code of Federal Regulations, Title 45, Part 46 (2009).

pared community colleges were to move toward greater use of data and research to improve student success. The center fielded an email survey of a national random sample of college administrators (111 responses out of a total sample of 189) and conducted case studies of 28 community colleges in 15 states. The study examined the research capacity in community colleges, how IR is used, and perceived barriers to the effective use of IR.

The following sections present our findings with respect to the typical staffing and governance of OIRs in colleges, the roles and responsibilities of these offices, and professional networks and organizations with which heads of OIRs are typically affiliated.

Staffing and Governance

Skills and Education Needed for Institutional Research Directors and Staff

Several respondents identified the importance of the IR director having graduate training or education, although most agreed that the position did not call for expertise in a particular discipline. The majority of the IR officers we interviewed had doctoral degrees, as did nearly 40 percent of the survey respondents in the CRCC survey. While the educational backgrounds of our respondents spanned a range of disciplines—economics, educational administration, education finance, human resource development, operations research, political science, social planning and policy—about a third of the CRCC respondents had advanced degrees in education and a quarter in social sciences.

Most of our respondents agreed that the director and staff of an OIR needed a mix of technical, interpersonal or social, and management skills: that it was not sufficient to simply be a good statistician or "data-cruncher." The staff—and the director, in particular—should have the skills to understand and communicate the numbers and relate them to the broader organizational or policy perspective of the institution. As one respondent noted, "You need the technical/research/analytic skills, but what is critical is knowing how to turn data into information." Staff clearly need to be experienced with data and programming, but beyond that, "They need to know how to write a report out of the data, tell you what the data mean, and explain it."

One IR director noted that, while statistical training helps, the office rarely conducts advanced statistical analysis. Directors need sufficient statistical skills to "hold our own" with statistics faculty or when presenting to the faculty senate, "but it's more important to have someone on your team that is a statistician." According to this respondent, the director needs analytic skills and knowledge of statistics and databases to effectively supervise quantitative analysts on his or her staff. "But the key to having an impact on campus is interpersonal skills, communication, to 'be able to be heard.'" A respondent from one of the professional organizations agreed, noting that presidents of community colleges tend to want good statisticians to crunch numbers, but the most important function of an IR officer is "the ability to generate trust, and it is the people skills that distinguish effective IR officers." Others emphasized the need for someone who understands the "big picture" or has a broader perspective of the institution and higher education.

In addition, many also noted the importance of IR directors possessing various types of experience: IR experience, experience with higher-education institutions, research and evaluation experience, planning experience (if strategic planning is part of the IR function), and experience in dealing with various constituencies ("political savvy").[2]

Governance and Communication

Respondents noted that the personality and interests of the person to whom the IR director reports significantly shapes what the OIR does, what its priorities are, how it is perceived by stakeholders in the institution, and the likelihood of results being valued and used. Most of the IR directors seemed to have indirect lines to the chancellor or president via a top-level administrator (e.g., vice president, vice chancellor, pro-

---

[2] The CRCC study noted that OIRs tended to be small and underfunded: About half the colleges surveyed employed just one or fewer full-time-equivalent staff members in their OIRs (Morest and Jenkins, 2007). In our interviews (our sample was predominantly large community colleges, with several colleges or campuses, and four-year institutions), OIRs were larger, ranging from four to 14 full-time-equivalent staff.

vost of academic affairs). The CRCC study also found that IR directors tended to fall into the middle management of a community college's organizational structure.

All our interviewees stressed the importance of having the chancellor or president's ear and reporting to a high-level person. One respondent noted that there were two sides to this: When the OIR director reports to the president, the benefit is that the OIR has the "weight" of the president behind it; the disadvantage is that people are less honest with the director. A respondent from a professional association noted that the only way for IR officers to be effective is to have a seat at the decisionmakers' table. The CRCC study concluded that the most successful OIRs that used student outcome data for planning and improvement were led by "an individual with experience and advanced training who is a full member of the college's leadership team, and they employ sufficient staff to conduct research above what is required for the purposes of compliance and accreditation" (Morest and Jenkins, 2007, p. 3).

Some respondents noted that IR has many constituents, which can be challenging. One rather humorously noted that, in her case, the president, provost, executive vice president, other vice presidents, and deans all felt that the office reported to them, which made the job a difficult balancing act. One respondent described potential "turf" issues arising from the fact that faculty had their own expert who assessed student learning outcomes and reported to the academic side while the OIR reported directly to the president. To avoid this, one institution set up a model in which the OIR reported to the "academic side" of the university because the vice chancellor for academic affairs felt that it was important for gaining credibility with faculty, who tended to be more responsive to information generated by an academic office.

Most IR officers serve on committees and governing bodies (for example, the steering committee for planning, data stewards committee, council of deans, or council of chairs) and participate in other meetings (for example, academic deans' monthly meetings), helping them anticipate data needs and provide data in a timely way to inform policy and decisions.

Objectivity was seen as critical to the effective functioning of the office. Thus, as one respondent noted, it is important to position the OIR as independent and not "in the pocket" of the person to whom it reports. The code of ethics established by AIR emphasizes that the institutional researcher should "approach all assignments with an unbiased attitude and strive to gather evidence fairly and accurately" (AIR, 2002). One respondent mentioned invoking this code in a situation in which the person to whom the OIR reported wanted to present data in a way that the respondent did not think was accurate.

Scope and Functions

OIRs vary widely in their scope of responsibilities. Offices associated with the four-year universities or the larger community colleges in our sample had fairly broad sets of functions. However, in a large college system, the central offices have more limited functions than the individual campus OIRs.

These functions include compliance reporting—described as "federal, state, accreditation, and grant reporting" by Morest and Jenkins (2007)—internal reporting, and research and analysis. To carry out these functions, OIRs are often involved in data warehousing or building data files from disparate sets of data. We describe these functions next.

Compliance Reporting

As Morest and Jenkins (2007, p. 8) note, "Much of the time of IR staff is devoted to reporting data to a variety of external stakeholders, especially state and federal government agencies." This includes basic data on enrollment, degree attainment, demographics, retention, transfer rates, job placement success, licensure pass rates, and student satisfaction. Often, many of these indicators are required for performance accountability reports to states and the federal government and have financial rewards or sanctions associated with them. Our respondents all emphasized that compliance reporting took up a substantial amount of time and that this had increased over the years. One institution estimated that it provided more than 50 annual reports to meet compliance requirements, and referred to it a "great burden." Morest and Jenkins (2007) reported that colleges do not perceive the time required to keep up with compliance reporting as well spent.

At one university, the OIR was responsible for leading the accreditation process, including conducting the self-study, providing documents to the accreditation association, and ensuring the university's compliance with accreditation requirements. At most other colleges and universities, the OIR played a more supportive role in the accreditation process: It contributed data but was not actually responsible for or leading the accreditation effort. One respondent mentioned that, originally, the OIR had been in charge of the accreditation effort, but this responsibility had devolved to another office; however, the OIR continued to provide considerable help with discipline accreditation by conducting surveys and focus groups for those departments.

Internal Reporting

Internal reporting or responding to various administrators for institutional and program data is the other major responsibility of OIRs. Some of these reports contain the same basic information as required for compliance reporting—for example, enrollments and degree attainment. The reports are produced regularly and are often made public (i.e., placed on websites). Some track trends over time, and some benchmark data against a set of peer institutions. Other reports track performance indicators tied to internal strategic plans; again, some of this is also done for compliance reporting. Most of the OIRs were not directly responsible for strategic planning but assisted in various ways, sitting on planning committees or playing a key role in providing data for their institutional "dashboards" and "balanced scorecards." Many respondents mentioned providing ad hoc reports based on requests from leadership and the need to be proactive in anticipating such requests because responding to requests from a variety of stakeholders took up so much time.

Research and Analysis

The CRCC study (Morest and Jenkins, 2007, p. 3) reported that the most successful OIRs (in the sense of being able to use data to manage and improve programs and services) "typically combine institutional research, planning, institutional effectiveness, and assessment into one department."

The majority of institutions reported conducting periodic surveys of students and faculty, such as entry and exit student surveys, student satisfaction surveys, course evaluations, and surveys of faculty regarding various academic and institutional issues. In one case, the OIR also conducted alumni and employer surveys.

A few institutions (generally, the four-year colleges and larger community colleges) reported participating in research and evaluation of programs or initiatives. These evaluations were often internal and intended to inform policy analysis. Examples of research and analysis activities undertaken by OIRs included evaluations for various grant programs or other special projects, tracking program outcomes, using evidence for program improvement, working with units to plan assessments and evaluations, providing guidance on survey development and implementation, and analyzing data to support key initiatives. One institution planned to ask its OIR to analyze the new full-time-equivalent funding model, class size, and faculty-student ratios.

Some OIRs in four-year institutions were also involved in assessing learning outcomes (for example, placement and exit testing), running the testing center, or collaborating with the campus teaching and learning center to look at student assessments using a value-added framework or address pedagogical questions through research.

A few of the OIR directors we interviewed mentioned participating in their institutional review boards. A director at one four-year institution mentioned training all OIR staff on the institutional review board requirements so that the staff could be helpful to faculty. In other institutions, this function was handled by other offices.

Data Warehousing and Building and Maintaining Data Files

Selecting or developing a data warehouse or information system seemed to be critical. One respondent strongly recommended that establishing a data warehouse to house data from disparate sources in one central database and implementing common definitions across courses, departments, and programs should be the first task of a new OIR.

Many respondents mentioned that it was essential for the OIR to have access to all relevant data on the institution. One college felt strongly that those building the data and those responsible for their accuracy and availability should be located in the same office. This institution merged its IR data staff in with its information technology staff to form a data-reporting team. At another institution, the IR director sat on several committees that directed the development of campus databases to ensure that she knew what was going on and could establish collaborative relationships.

Three other themes emerged from our interviews. First, many noted that data needed to be maintained in ways that allowed for easy and quick access, because IR offices generally get requests that require quick turnaround. Some expressed a commitment to ensuring that these data are accessible to individuals outside the OIR, thus lowering the burden on IR staff to continuously respond to requests for data. Second, ensuring data access also necessitates a clear understanding and delineation of rules concerning who has permission to interact with information technology and how to ensure proper protections and security. Third, several respondents identified the importance ensuring the accuracy and consistency of IR data. One respondent emphasized the importance of using common definitions to enable accurate comparisons across semesters, courses, or years. Something as simple as the number of students enrolled in a course could differ if the data are pulled at different points in time. An interviewee from one large four-year institution described cleaning data as a major function of the OIR and noted that this is particularly important when data are being merged from multiple databases.

Examples of How Institutional Research Reporting Has Influenced Decisionmaking

When asked, many respondents provided examples of ways in which the reporting of IR data has influenced decisions or practices in their institution:

- Data from a student survey highlighting student dissatisfaction with pre-major advising and school-related stress in the first year of veterinary school led to changes in that program.
- Data showing the disconnect between plans for a new college of education building and its proposed use led to changes in the planned building.
- Analysis showing that grade point average in a student's first year is a good predictor of retention led to investments in tutoring, labs, and other approaches to help raise students' averages; this, in turn, increased retention.
- Research on the effect of financial aid on retention and the effectiveness of certain programs aimed at retention led to changes in the allocation of financial aid and the structure of the programs.

A respondent from one institution reported an innovative approach to systematically examining how data were being used throughout the system. The OIR developed a report template that asks the disciplines and service areas whether they are meeting outcome goals, how they are measuring them, and how they are using the results of their assessments. The data are submitted to IR staff, who present the results of the analysis and help the departments understand how to use the data more effectively to improve. The OIR at that institution surveys the departments annually to determine how they have used the data and to identify any data that have "shocked" them into thinking differently.

Networking and Professional Associations

All our respondents stressed the importance of networking and participating in professional associations. The most frequently mentioned professional association was AIR. Almost all the respondents had been active participants or leaders in AIR at some point in their careers. The overwhelming majority believed that membership in AIR was very valuable for their work and for being ethical practitioners (several mentioned the AIR code of ethics). One institution called it "a wonderful resource," while another mentioned that it facilitates collaboration, sharing of best practices, and "helps you answer questions about thorny issues."

Many also highly recommended participation in regional or state AIR organizations and noted that the Southern Association of Institutional Research, which would be a natural fit for METC, is very strong and active. These regional associations are, as one respondent put it, "a more humane size, better for networking."

Respondents also described various other associations and organizations that might be relevant to an OIR, depending on its scope, functions, and the type of institution. For offices involved in research and evaluation, three prominent professional associations were mentioned as helpful:

- the Association for the Study of Higher Education, which "promotes collaboration among its members and others engaged in the study of higher education through research, conferences, and publications" (ASHE, undated).
- the American Educational Research Association, which "is concerned with improving the educational process by encouraging scholarly inquiry related to education and evaluation and by promoting the dissemination and practical application of research results" (AERA, 2010).
- the American Evaluation Association, an "international professional association of evaluators devoted to the application and exploration of program evaluation, personnel evaluation, technology, and many other forms of evaluation. Evaluation involves assessing the strengths and weaknesses of programs, policies, personnel, products, and organizations to improve their effectiveness" (AEA, undated).

For offices involved in strategic research, one respondent recommended the Society for College and University Planning, a professional association devoted to improving integrated planning for higher education and offering knowledge communities and several online resources.

Institutions belonged to various other associations that represent higher-education institutions (such as the American Association of Community Colleges and the Coalition of Urban and Metropolitan Universities) or associations that promoted innovation in community colleges (such as the League for Innovation in Community Colleges). One respondent highly recommended the latter, saying that it was about sharing best practices and focused on helping community colleges fulfill their mission. As such, it had a broader focus than simply IR. Some of the colleges participated in various reform initiatives, including Achieving the Dream, or state advisory task forces that focused on improving community colleges' data systems.

Overall, our respondents stressed the importance of networking, calling it "critical" to making the office more effective and providing professional growth and learning opportunities for the director and staff.

Advice or Recommendations for METC

Respondents noted several challenges to the effective functioning of an OIR and, based on their experiences, proffered advice and recommendations for METC when setting up a new OIR:

Determine the scope and functions of the office. METC leadership will need to establish and prioritize the work of the OIR in terms of data management, internal reporting, external reporting, accreditation, strategic planning, and other activities. One of the most important tasks is to establish a common terminology and timing for data collection.

Organize data management and technology. METC's OIR will need to determine where the necessary data currently exist, in what form, and who has access to those data. It will also need to develop an organized process to collect and warehouse them in one central location, with particular attention to data quality, access, and protection.

Determine the structure and governance of the office. Where an OIR is located within a broader organization or institution matters. Reporting and governance arrangements tend to shape what OIRs do and the types of questions they answer. The OIR needs to be located fairly high up in the hierarchy of METC to ensure that IR is taken seriously and that the director has credibility and the authority to access the needed data. Sitting at the table with decisionmakers is important: It helps the OIR position its data correctly and inform higher-level policy and improvement.

Hire the right staff. Ensuring a skilled staff means assembling individuals who have both technical skills (statistics, information technology, programming) and broader enterprise knowledge, communication abilities, and interpersonal skills—particularly in how to turn data into information and convey its meaning. The latter was seen as particularly important for a director of IR, whereas the former were cited as important skills for OIR staff. Experience in the higher-education field was also seen as critical. Credibility and trust comes not only with experience but also credentials. Political skills were also viewed as key by some respondents.

Finally, it is equally important to have an adequate staff to meet the demands of various stakeholders. Capacity constraints affect both the ability to collect, maintain, and analyze data and the quality of the reports produced from these data.

Establish collaborative relationships with other METC departments. It is important to extend opportunities for all concerned stakeholders to provide input into the process and to get their buy-in. One respondent said, "Don't stay in your office. Interact, go to meetings, sit on committees—be proactive." Participating in institutional committees is important for understanding institutional and programmatic needs and priorities, anticipating data needs and emerging issues, and being proactive in providing the needed data. To minimize the burden of constantly responding to data requests, the system should be made more transparent by putting reports on the web or making data accessible to programs and faculty. As with other METC departments, it is important for OIR staff to be active members of professional associations and to network, so travel must be built into the budget. This would help encourage the personal and professional growth of the director and staff and further their learning about best practices.

CHAPTER FIVE

Lessons Learned from Organizations with Training Missions Similar to That of METC

This chapter describes research and evaluation efforts undertaken by organizations that have missions similar to that of METC to draw out lessons of relevance to METC and provide concrete examples of the types of research and evaluation being undertaken by these organizations. These organizations include the following:

- corporate universities that are separate entities within companies and primarily responsible for the development and implementation of training programs for members of the organization (Meister, 1994)
- DMETA, set up by the United Kingdom's MoD in 2003 as an executive agency to (among other objectives) deliver appropriate medical and military training and education to the three military services to meet operational requirement (DMETA, 2008)[1]
- other federal agencies with a focus on training and development.

METC closely resembles a corporate university in that it was set up to provide consolidated medical education and training to Army, Navy, and Air Force medical enlisted personnel to support the mission of the MHS. As such, lessons drawn from corporate universities would be useful as METC goes forward.

At the same time, METC is a direct counterpart of DMETA, with the same training mission. It will be considerably larger in terms

---

[1] In April 2008, DMETA was brought under the newly established Joint Medical Command, which has broader responsibilities than DMETA.

of average daily student attendance and total number of faculty but narrower in scope in the sense that METC's responsibility is limited to enlisted medical personnel training.

Finally, METC could benefit from best practices in performance measurement and evaluation in the federal sector and could learn from the experiences of other federal agencies that have made considerable investments in training and development.

Corporate Universities

Allen (2002, p. 9) defines a corporate university as "an educational entity that is a strategic tool designed to assist its parent organization in achieving its mission by conducting activities that foster individual and organizational learning, knowledge and wisdom." In that sense, a corporate university is different from a training department, which simply conducts training. A corporate university must be strategic in intent and activities. We also note that corporate universities do not exist only in corporations; they are found in governmental agencies and not-for-profit companies as well.[2]

Although corporate universities differ in scope and function, measurement and evaluation of program effectiveness is always a key component. Studies comparing the experiences of best-practice organizations reveal that there is no single "correct" model of evaluation. (The section "Evaluation," later in this chapter, reviews commonly used models of evaluation along with GAO guidelines for conducting evaluations of training programs.) However, the literature does reveal some

---

[2]   Allen and McGee (2004) further explicate three key aspects of this definition. First, the focus of the corporate university is strategic, which implies that learning is valued only insofar as it contributes to organizational goals (as opposed to learning for its own sake, which is valued in traditional universities). Second, the corporate university aims to promote both individual and organizational learning. Third, the emphasis on "wisdom" means that the corporate university is interested in the intelligent application of knowledge. They note, "The organization does not benefit if knowledge is acquired but not used" (Allen and McGee, 2004, p. 83).

common themes regarding the importance and structure of program evaluation in corporate universities.

First, corporate training leaders devote significant resources and attention to evaluation. Organizations with strong reputations for training, such as Motorola, AT&T, Microsoft, and Marriott, have full-scale evaluation units within their training departments (Geber, 1995). Dixon (1996) notes that even when corporations such as Motorola or IBM outsource the actual delivery of training, they consistently retain in-house evaluation of training.

Second, best-practice organizations seem to build evaluation into training programs early by devoting considerable attention to evaluation issues in the program development and planning phase. Thinking about evaluation and measurement as part of the planning process can also help training developers sharpen their focus and define their objectives. As Allen and McGee (2004, p. 86) point out,

> What to measure is simply the answer to the question, "What are we trying to accomplish?" The close connection between goals and measurement reinforces the notion that measurement is part of the planning process, not something considered after the fact.

Third, best-practice organizations emphasize a focus on the customer in their evaluation efforts. (A "customer" in this sense might be the consumer of the organization's ultimate product or service, but the term could also include internal customers who receive the work product or have other relationships with trainees.) Evaluators in these corporations consult with customers—broadly construed—to determine their requirements and to learn which standards to set and what to measure (Dixon, 1996). Trainers and evaluators are typically not in a position to understand "bottom-line" needs on their own, so collaboration with others helps them understand what is important at the organizational level (Watson, 1998).

Fourth, organizations identified as leaders in training evaluation tend to emphasize the concept of "evidence" over that of "proof." As we show later, there are a number of methodological challenges related to measuring change and attributing effects to single programs;

some evidence suggests that such challenges may discourage managers from evaluating training if they feel that "proof" is required but do not perceive it as possible (Honeycutt and Stevenson, 1989; Camp, Blanchard, and Huszczo, 1986). Instead, as Dixon (1996) notes, "Best-practice companies seem less concerned with collecting irrefutable evidence than with determining whether the desired result was obtained." Determining precise cause-and-effect relationships in the face of so many external factors that cannot be controlled may be impossible, but for the purposes of program evaluation and improvement, showing a relationship and evidence that training made a difference seems to be enough for many best-practice organizations (Geber, 1995; Watson, 1998).

Finally, evaluation in best-practice organizations is focused on program improvement. Much of the literature on training evaluation seems oriented toward teaching trainers to collect evidence to help them justify their programs to higher-ups or to maintain their departmental budgets. Corporations that use training evaluations most effectively, however, have evaluators who are interested in the broader picture of organizational improvement, rather than interorganizational turf wars (Allen and McGee, 2004; Dixon, 1996). The purpose of a corporate university is to help its parent organization achieve its mission; as such, it is important to rely on mission-based metrics that are organization-specific when judging the overall effectiveness of the corporate university.

Defence Medical Education and Training Agency

The UK's Defence Medical Services, headed jointly by the Deputy Chief of the Defence Staff (Health) and the Surgeon General, was recently reorganized.[3] It currently consists of (1) the Defence Medi-

---

[3] This section draws heavily from research conducted by RAND colleagues Amanda Scoggins and Hans Pung as part of the overall METC project. The findings were presented to METC's executive integrated process team in the form of an internal memorandum, *Joint Defence Medical Education and Training: A Case Study of UK's Defence Medical Education and Training Agency*, in October 2007.

cal Services Department, which is the headquarters for the Defence Medical Services and provides strategic direction to ensure delivery of defense medical outputs, and (2) the Joint Medical Command, a joint service organization charged with providing secondary care personnel to meet requirements for operational deployments,[4] supporting frontline units by educating and training medical personnel through DMETA, and providing dental services to personnel through the Defence Dental Services.[5] In addition, the three armed medical services—the Royal Naval Medical Service, the Army Medical Services, and the Royal Air Force Medical Services—are responsible for delivering primary health care to their respective services and for providing the required medical support in operations.

As noted in the introduction to this chapter, DMETA was originally established as a triservice, multisite organization and an executive agency of MoD and folded into the Joint Medical Command in 2008. Two of the principal objectives of DMETA are to provide medical, dental, and military education and training according to specified statutory, professional, and military standards to personnel in the Defence Medical Services and elsewhere and to develop training and training policy in response to changes in doctrine, medical practice, research and development, and equipment acquisition so as to teach best practices that are appropriate to the military environment (DMETA, 2003, 2008).

Training Conducted by DMETA for Allied Health Professionals

British military service training is conducted in three phases. Phase 1 training is delivered within the single service context and includes courses that are military-specific and that all professions must complete. Phase 2 training courses are profession- or role-specific and may be carried out in the MoD or single-service arena. Phase 3 training is

---

[4] Secondary care personnel are those who are generally not the first point-of-contact with medical patients. Instead, they provide more comprehensive or specialized medical services for the British Armed Forces.

[5] The Defence Dental Services came under the Joint Medical Command's umbrella in mid-2009.

subsequent training and education delivered as continuing professional development and is typically undertaken to achieve a higher professional rank (i.e., promotion) or to gain employment-specific expertise.

DMETA is responsible for most Phase 2 and Phase 3 training delivered to the Defence Medical Services. Some of this training is delivered in military establishments or in partnership with other providers, including universities. DMETA Phase 3 courses may entail joint or single-service training.

Similar to METC's goal, DMETA provides training to allied health professionals (e.g., radiographers, operating department technicians) and combat medical technicians or medical assistants. The former are either direct entrants or join their service untrained before receiving training at the Defence School of Health Care Studies, a DMETA unit, which is affiliated with the University of Birmingham and Birmingham City University. These latter personnel, the largest group in the Defence Medical Services, do not require formal qualifications to enter the services. Instead, this group receives general training through the Common Core Course (approximately 20 weeks), the largest-throughput Phase 2 training course. The Common Core Course includes 12 weeks of classroom training, six weeks of a clinical attachment, and two weeks of assessment. In addition to the Common Core Course, service-specific training is undertaken to account for the difference in environments encountered by British Army, Royal Navy, and Royal Air Force personnel.

DMETA also administers follow-on courses, such as Advanced Military Acute Care for Medical Assistants and Medical Administration and Battlefield Advanced Trauma Life Support. There are approximately 80 joint Defence Medical Services courses.

DMETA's Approach to Training

DMETA's approach to the training process follows the Defence Systems Approach to Training (DSAT) quality standard, which sets out the strategic principles to be applied to all individual training provided by, or on behalf of, MoD. The fundamental principles of the DSAT quality standard are as follows (UK Ministry of Defence, 2003):

The aim of training is to prepare personnel for their current or future operational or workplace role.

Training provided by, or on behalf of, the MoD must have a clearly identified MoD sponsor.

Training must be formally authorised and resourced.

Training provided by, or on behalf of, the MoD is to be derived from an analysis of the operational/workplace requirements.

Training is designed to achieve training objectives based on the results of the needs analysis.

Training objectives are to be endorsed by the sponsor.

Training objectives are to be achieved by the most efficient and effective use of resources.

Training must have an evaluation strategy.

There must be an evaluation of the efficiency and effectiveness of the analysis, design and delivery of training in meeting the operational/business requirements in accordance with the Evaluation Strategy.

The currency of training activities is to be maintained by applying the results of evaluation.

All activities related to training must comply with all relevant extant legislation (e.g. Health and Safety, Equal Opportunities, Data Protection Act etc).

The DSAT espouses a systematic process for developing and delivering training, as illustrated by Figure 5.1. In general, the DSAT follows a cyclical approach, but each stage is iterative. Initially, there is a needs analysis to determine the training that is required. That training is then designed and developed in alignment with the standard. It is then delivered to the target audience. Upon completion of the training, both the training deliverer and the customer follow validation procedures to ensure that the training is delivering its desired effect. Continuous evaluation surrounds the entire process to allow adjustments to be made as needed. Both the DSAT model and the fundamental prin-

Figure 5.1
The Defence Systems Approach to Training Model

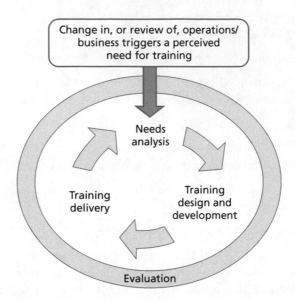

SOURCE: UK Ministry of Defence, 2003, p. 6, Diagram 1.1. Used in accordance with guidelines governing Crown Copyright.
RAND *MG981-5.1*

ciples emphasize the importance of building in evaluation and feed-back to improve the training.

Evaluation

DSAT uses evaluation to monitor the impact of training and assess outcomes, including whether the training was effective and efficient and how it contributed to the achievement of the organization's goals and targets. The DSAT quality standard originally identified six stages of a training evaluation; the first two were (1) produce a training evaluation strategy and (2) identify training needs. These first two stages were subsequently dropped; the current model's four stages resemble the stages of a traditional training evaluation model, such as the "balanced scorecard" discussed in the next section. The four stages of the DSAT are as follows:

1. Measure the immediate reaction of the individual through an after-action review.
2. Measure the learning transfer achieved by the training activity.
3. Measure changes in the behavior of the individual as a result of the training activity and how well enhancement of knowledge, skills, or attitudes has prepared the individual for his or her role.
4. Measure the contribution of the training to the achievement of business or operational goals (UK Ministry of Defence, 2003).

According to the DSAT quality standard, all training should be subject to the first two evaluation stages. It also states the application of the third and fourth stages must consider the actual or perceived impact of the training activity on operational performance; the cost of the evaluation compared to the realized, potential, or perceived benefits of the training activity; and the utility of the evaluation's outputs. The evaluation strategy includes the targets and performance indicators that are pertinent to training activities and must involve all relevant stakeholders at the appropriate management level. In practice, stages 1 and 2 are achieved by conducting internal validation (InVal) within the training delivery units in accordance with the DMETA InVal policy. Stages 3 and 4 are achieved by conducting external validation (ExVal), the responsibility for which lies with the customer agents. However, DMETA has taken a more proactive stance and coordinates the ExVal across the three services in accordance with the DMETA ExVal policy agreed to by the services. DMETA also implemented an "early warning feedback" form of ExVal (stage 3) to identify and inform the requirement for a more rigorous and full ExVal or evaluation (stage 4) of the training. The results of this full ExVal are fed back into the system and used to check the accuracy of operational performance statements and to prove that the training being delivered meets the operational requirements of the services.

Performance Targets

The Defence Health Programme uses a "balanced scorecard" for assessing a department's performance against objectives (UK Ministry of Defence, 2005, p. 9). The scorecard focuses on the following four questions:

- *Purpose:* Is the department fit for today's challenges and ready for tomorrow's tasks?
- *Enabling processes:* Is the department a high-performing organization?
- *Resources:* Is the department using its resources to best effect?
- *Future capabilities:* Is the department building for future success?

It outlines several performance indicators and associated targets in each of these areas that DMETA is required to report to the Deputy Chief of the Defence Staff (Health). Performance targets are proposed by DMETA, discussed with the Deputy Chief of the Defence Staff (Health), and then forwarded for approval by ministers. Performance indicators are discussed, developed, and agreed to internally at DMETA.

Table 5.2 presents DMETA's performance against key targets for 2007–2008.

Federal Agencies and the Push Toward Performance Measurement

The GAO undertook a series of studies in early 2000 of how federal agencies were attempting to transform their cultures and position themselves to face the challenges of the 21st century. In their transformation efforts, agencies were investing resources, including time and money, in training and developing employees and providing them with the information, skills, and competencies they needed to work effectively in a rapidly changing and complex environment. The GAO review highlighted human capital shortfalls in agencies' efforts to train and develop their workforces, including insufficient training for employees who lacked needed skills and competencies and duplicative or unco-ordinated efforts within and across agencies. The Office of Personnel Management reported that only about half of the federal employees responding to the 2002 Federal Human Capital Survey were satisfied

Table 5.2
DMETA's Performance Against Key Targets

Key Target	2007–2008	
	Target	Achieved
1. Deployable personnel	100%	100%
To meet the requirements of the commanders in chief for secondary care personnel under DMETA command for operational deployments		
2. Individual military continuation training	90%	91%
To ensure that 90% of all DMETA personnel, whose medical category permits, achieve their service's annual mandatory individual military training		
3. Medical professional and career training		
a. To provide initial training (Phase 2) that meets the requirements, professional standards, and timescales defined by the services	> 95%	96.9%
b. To provide career, professional, and continuation training (Phase 3) that meets the requirements, professional standards, and timescales defined by the services and the statutory requirements of the relevant national bodies	> 95%	98.9%
4. Efficiency	2.25:1	2.4:1
To reduce the ratio of personnel engaged in support activities to personnel engaged in direct activities		
5. Customer focus	62–65	63
To maintain the Customer Confidence Index score within a stated range		
6. Harmony/separated service	100%	99.75%
To ensure compliance with the services' harmony guidelines for all deployable personnel under DMETA's command		

SOURCE: DMETA, 2008, pp. 12–14. Adapted in accordance with guidelines governing Crown Copyright.

with the training that they received for their current jobs. The GAO report concluded,

> Thoroughly assessing their training and development activities represents a comprehensive first step that federal agencies can take toward identifying opportunities to redirect and intensify their efforts to promote employee learning within the organization. (GAO, 2004c, p. 2)

More recently, the Obama administration signaled its commitment to performance measurement and program evaluation by emphasizing these activities in the "Analytical Perspectives" section of the FY 2011 President's budget. Indeed, the budget includes a separate chapter called "Program Evaluation" (see Office of Management and Budget, 2010), which clearly outlines the administration's position:

> Empirical evidence is an essential ingredient for assessing whether Government programs are achieving their intended outcomes. . . .
>
> A central pillar of good government is a culture where answering such questions is a fundamental part of program design and where agencies have the capacity to use evidence to invest more in what works and less in what does not. (Office of Management and Budget, 2010, p. 91)

The chapter also points out that one of the challenges in evidence-based policymaking is that evaluations are often added as an afterthought, after programs are designed, making rigorous evaluations difficult. It outlines a three-tiered approach that provides additional resources for programs that generate results backed by strong evidence:

> Organizations will know that to be considered for significant funding, they must provide credible evaluation results that show promise, and before that evidence is available, to be ready to subject their models to analysis. . . .
>
> By instilling a culture of learning into Federal programs, the Administration can build knowledge so that spending decisions are based not only on good intentions, but also on strong evidence, so that carefully targeted investments will produce results. (Office of Management and Budget, 2010, p. 92)

Lessons Learned from Other Government Agencies

GAO Assessment of Five Federal Agencies. The GAO recommends that organizations continually look to other agencies to identify innovative approaches that may be useful in their own training and development efforts. "Benchmarking is a technique that can help agencies determine who is the very best, who sets the standards, and what that standard is" (GAO, 2004c, p. 75). The GAO, in an earlier report (2004a), shared experiences and lessons learned from the design of effective training and development programs in five federal agencies: the U.S. Army Corps of Engineers, DoD; the U.S. Fish and Wildlife Service, U.S. Department of the Interior; the Internal Revenue Service, U.S. Department of the Treasury; the Office of Personnel Management; and the VHA, U.S. Department of Veterans Affairs (VA). With respect to evaluation, the GAO noted that while the five agencies relied primarily on standard end-of-course evaluations, they had begun or planned to use more comprehensive and sophisticated techniques for measuring the extent to which the training and development programs increased employees' knowledge and skills and enhanced individual and organizational performance. Examples of these techniques included pre- and post testing, tracking changes in individual and program performance, and some limited use of return-on-investment (ROI) analyses (GAO, 2004a). Some of the lessons learned by the five agencies in designing methods to evaluate training and development programs included the following:

> Incorporate appropriate aspects of the evaluation approach when designing training and development programs by specifying what results are expected to better ensure the availability and use of quality performance data.

> Consider new approaches for collecting and analyzing performance data with the aim of increasing the quality and quantity of training evaluation feedback.

> Plan for the use of multiple data types and sources to provide a balanced approach in assessing the effectiveness of training and development programs.

> Take into account all relevant factors for determining the costs of a training and development program to better ascertain whether it is cost effective in relation to benefits achieved. (GAO, 2004a, pp. 4–5)

We now turn our focus on the VHA and what METC could learn from that organization.

Veterans Health Administration. As part of the larger overall project that RAND undertook for METC, we were asked to examine how different sectors developed health care leaders for executive positions. During the course of that research, we conducted a case study of the VHA because it was similar in scope to the MHS and the two had close relationships and ties. With more than 235,000 employees, the VHA is the third-largest civilian employer in the federal government and one of the largest providers of health care in the world. It is also the nation's largest integrated health care delivery system and provides care through a system of 21 Veterans Integrated Service Networks (VISNs) distributed throughout the United States.

The results of our study, documented in Kirby et al. (2010) show that over the past several years, the VHA has spent considerable time and effort transforming itself into a high-performing learning organization, and its workforce development and succession plan has been recognized by the Office of Personnel Management as a federal best practice (VA, 2009). A VHA senior leader noted recently that that the organization is undergoing significant transformation under the new VA and VHA leadership, including the launching of a comprehensive human capital initiative to make the VA a "veteran- and people-centric, results-oriented, and forward-looking organization."[6] As part of this effort, the VHA is evaluating its current development programs to ensure that they meet and further the goals of the new leadership.

For the purposes of this monograph, we want to highlight some features of the VHA and recommend that METC develop a collaborative relationship with that organization to draw lessons learned regarding the design and implementation of strategic training and development efforts.

First, the VHA has established the National Center for Organizational Development (NCOD), a central office that measures and

---

[6] Personal communication, April 4, 2010.

monitors the organizational health of the VHA. While an NCOD-like organization would be more appropriate at the MHS-level, we believe that many of the activities and approaches used by NCOD would have relevance for METC. For example, NCOD conducts, analyzes, and interprets the VHA's All Employee Survey and then provides customized feedback to networks and facilities.[7] The survey has a very high response rate—76 percent in 2007 and 73 percent in 2008. It has three components: (1) the Job Satisfaction Index, a 13-dimensional scale that measures employees' individual satisfaction with key job features; (2) the Organizational Assessment Inventory, a 20-dimensional scale that measures employees' perceptions of conditions in their immediate work group; and (3) a culture section, a set of questions that measure employees' perceptions of the general atmosphere at their facility overall and maps to four dimensions. The data are analyzed at the network, facility, and (where possible) work-group level; these analyses show longitudinal trends within the unit of analysis (for example, for a particular VISN or facility) and a comparison with overall VHA averages, including the statistical significance of the differences. The NCOD staff prepare and present briefings to each network and facility and help interpret differences and trends. They advise the network or facility to focus on practical versus statistical significance (i.e., differences that are large enough to matter substantively) and to give greater weight to patterns rather than one-off findings. Feedback is a critical element of the VHA's quality-improvement plan. Trends and comparative standings are tracked and highlighted. The findings are reported to senior leadership and taken seriously in performance evaluations.

---

[7]   NCOD has several other functions. For example, it conducts 360- and 180-degree assessments of individuals and is responsible for feedback and assessment of the critical skills of leader candidates. It develops customized assessment instruments for network and facility leaders and conducts site visits to places struggling with issues of organizational health. In addition, it offers interventions to improve organizational health. One such initiative is called Civility, Respect, and Engagement in the Workplace, which was developed in-house. Respondents noted that this intervention has improved the culture and working relationships among the teams and facilities that have adopted it.

Second, the 2007 VHA strategic plan emphasizes the continuous assessment, feedback, and redesign for all VHA training and development programs:

> Workforce succession program evaluation is a part of the annual strategic planning process and an integral part of the operation of each individual program. Programs are reviewed within the context of the overall workforce analyses and specific plans and needs identified by each VISN. Recommendations for program changes are then included in the update process for the national plan. VHA developed a general model for program evaluation and each program design incorporates the appropriate evaluation methodologies consistent with this overall evaluation model. (VA, 2007, p. 14)

One respondent interviewed for our study noted the change that had occurred in the VHA over the past eight to ten years with respect to making program evaluation a central piece of every program:

> [T]he last five years we have been establishing a . . . stronger measurement function. . . . It's not just about making sure that we . . . "do evaluation" but . . . how are we driving and managing the data that we're collecting and then using it to make better program decisions. . . . That's going to be our focus for 2009 moving forward and upgrading our systems and really taking a more strategic look at how we use the data for improvement.

The VHA uses the Kirkpatrick model for program evaluation with standardized data-collection instruments so that it can establish consistency across programs and track changes in programs' reported effectiveness over time. (The Kirkpatrick model and levels are discussed in the section "Evaluation," later in this chapter.) Some programs get higher-level evaluations; for example, evaluators will interview supervisors to determine the effect of the program on performance, jobs, and the organization. For a small portion of its programs, VHA has begun to implement Level 5 evaluations to "not just measure satisfaction with learning but really look at the transference of learning into performance and actual practice on the job, and then linking that to business outcomes and return on investment," as one respondent noted. Because these evaluations tend to be very resource-intensive and may take longer to conduct, the VHA selects only a few programs for Level 5 evaluations.

GAO's Framework for Assessing Strategic Training and Development Efforts in the Federal Government

Given the ongoing and increasing emphasis on performance measurement and evaluation, METC needs to make evaluation an integral part of its training efforts and collect the evidence necessary to show that its programs are furthering the mission of the MHS and DoD—and doing so in a cost-effective manner.[8] This can be greatly facilitated by adopting the strategic framework outlined by the GAO (2004c) in response to a perceived need for a systematic yet flexible guide to help federal agencies in planning, designing, implementing, and evaluating effective training and development programs. The GAO developed this framework based on consultations with government officials and experts in the private sector, nonprofit sector, and academia; an examination of laws and regulations governing training and development in the federal government; and a review of the relevant literature. In what follows, we first outline the four components of the training and development process and then discuss the fourth component— evaluation—in greater detail.

Components of the Training and Development Process

The GAO's training and development process consists of four inter-related components, as shown in Figure 5.2. These components are familiar to any agency involved in providing training. What is most important to our discussion is the emphasis at each step that the programs be strategic in nature and designed to assist the agency in achiev-

---

[8]   This section draws primarily on GAO (2004c).

Figure 5.2
Four Components of the GAO's Training and Development Process

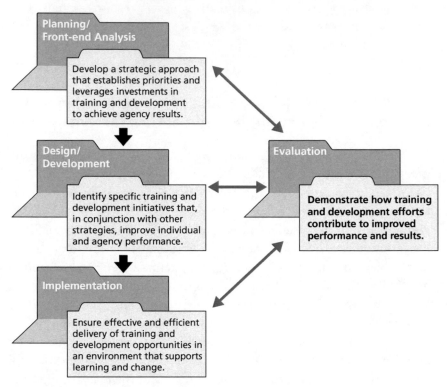

SOURCE: Source: GAO, 2004c, p. 4, Figure 2.
RAND *MG981-5.2*

ing its mission by improving individual and, ultimately, organizational performance (GAO, 2004c, p. 2).

In particular, the GAO highlights the importance of integrating evaluation into each step of the process. The report offers a clear rationale for doing so:

> It is increasingly important for agencies to be able to evaluate their training and development programs and demonstrate how these efforts help develop employees and improve the agencies' performance. In the past, agencies have primarily focused on activities or processes (such as number of training participants, courses, or hours) and did not collect information on how training and

development efforts contributed to improved performance, reduced costs, or a greater capacity to meet new and emerging transformation challenges. Because the evaluation of training and development programs can aid decision makers in managing scarce resources, agencies need to develop evaluation processes that systematically track the cost and delivery of training and development efforts and assess the benefits of these efforts. . . .

It is important to note that the federal government is increasingly moving toward connecting resources with results, and this is no less the case for training and development efforts than for other agency programs. . . . The bottom line is that agencies need credible information on how training and development programs affect organizational performance. Decision makers will likely want to compare the performance of these programs with that of other programs, and programs lacking outcome metrics will be unable to demonstrate how they contribute to results. (GAO, 2004c, p. 8)

Evaluation

The GAO framework lists several key questions that can help an agency develop and implement strategic evaluations that incorporate best practices in the field. Here, we reframe these questions as recommendations for agencies when designing and implementing evaluations:

- Systematically plan for and evaluate the effectiveness of training and development efforts.
- Use appropriate analytical approaches to assess training and development programs.
- Include a broad array of performance data (including qualitative and quantitative measures) to assess the results achieved through training and development efforts.
- Incorporate evaluation feedback into the planning, design, and implementation of training and development efforts.
- Incorporate different perspectives (including those of line managers and staff, customers, and experts in such areas as finance, information, and human capital management) in assessing the impact of training on performance.

- Track the cost and delivery of training and development programs.
- Assess the benefits achieved through training and development programs, and determine whether and when the benefits outweigh the projected costs through an ROI calculation.
- Compare training investments, methods, and outcomes with those of other organizations to identify innovative approaches or lessons learned.

Traditional training evaluations have often used fairly simple indicators of inputs and outputs that can be readily quantified. However, to assess how the training contributes to the accomplishment of agency objectives and goals, additional measures are needed. The GAO recommends developing a data-collection and -analysis plan that clearly outlines the goals that the program is expected to achieve and agreed-upon measures that can help determine the progress being made toward these goals. It also recommends adopting a balanced, multilevel approach to evaluation that incorporates various perspectives and provides a variety of data with which to measure the impact of the training on the organization. Agencies should use a balanced approach that relies on both quantitative data (for example, productivity or output, quality, costs, and time) and qualitative data (for example, employee satisfaction, managers' views on the extent to which employees transferred what they learned to their jobs, and feedback from customers) to assess the results of the training program.

One commonly accepted training evaluation model is the Kirkpatrick model, first articulated in the late 1950s. Although a handful of authors have recently critiqued the model as lacking theoretical grounding (see Wang and Spitzer, 2005) or have pointed out that it is a descriptive taxonomy rather than a method or operational tool (see Geber, 1995), it continues to dominate the training evaluation literature, in part because it is, as Kirkpatrick himself notes, "simple and practical." Kirkpatrick (1959) posits four stages or levels of training evaluations:

- Level 1: reactions
- Level 2: learning

- Level 3: behavior
- Level 4: results.[9]

A Level 1 evaluation focuses on *reactions*, or how trainees feel about the training. This is the most common form of training evaluation and is typically conducted using post-training surveys. The assumption is that negative reactions to training often indicate a lack of effort and motivation that will affect learning, while positive reactions indicate a more salutary mindset for learning (Leach and Liu, 2003; Lupton, Weiss, and Peterson, 1999). Reaction data can also provide useful formative information about the relevance of training, areas of participant confusion, the appropriateness of the content, the extent of trainee engagement, and so on. However, as Lupton, Weiss, and Peterson (1999) note, reactions can be easily influenced by such factors as location, setting, personality, and the timing of surveys immediately after the event (i.e., "halo" effect), which may be peripheral to the actual effectiveness of the training.

A Level 2 evaluation examines the *learning* that results from training, which may include both the acquisition and retention of knowledge, skills, or attitudes. Measurement requires an assessment of some sort and may involve determining gain scores from pre-post tests.

A Level 3 evaluation focuses on the extent to which learning is reflected in *job-related behavior*, or "transfer of learning." Some sort of change in behavior is the goal of most training programs. As Allen and McGee (2004, p. 84) note, "Learning without behavior change is merely learning for its own sake, which is generally not the goal of corporate universities." More than reactions or learning, the trainee's ability to transfer learning into behavior is often dependent on conditions that may not be within the control of the trainers, such as aspects

---

[9] The model is presumed to be hierarchical in nature, meaning that improvements at one level are believed to directly affect the next level: Positive reactions to training promote better learning, better learning results in better behavior, and better behavior leads to better organizational results. While some research has supported these relationships (see Alliger et al., 1997; Leach and Liu, 2003; and Warr and Bunce, 1995), other studies cast doubt on the extent to which results at one level are predictive of changes at higher levels (see Mann and Robertson, 1996; and Campion and Campion, 1987).

of the trainee's work environment, the trainee's knowledge of how to translate learning into behavior and available supports to aid in that process, and the trainee's motivation—both intrinsic and extrinsic—to change his or her behavior (Leach and Liu, 2003; Lupton, Weiss, and Peterson, 1999). Measurement of behavior is generally more challenging than measurement of reactions or learning. Examples of measurement strategies include trainee self-reports, direct observations, 360-degree assessments (feedback from trainees' supervisors, peers, and subordinates), and analysis of logbooks or other job-related artifacts (Leach and Liu, 2003; Geber, 1995; Mann and Robertson, 1996).

A Level 4 evaluation addresses *outcomes*, which are usually considered to be organization-level concerns. While they are sometimes focused on final, bottom-line outcomes, such as profits or revenue, Level 4 indicators can be anything of importance to the organization, such as customer satisfaction or employee turnover—or, in a health care context, improved patient outcomes. Although a Level 4 evaluation could require new data collection, a number of authors note that organizations often are already producing vast amounts of data that can be used for evaluation purposes (Geber, 1995; Watson, 1998). Organization-level outcomes are generally influenced by a host of factors extraneous to the training program, which makes the attribution of observed changes extremely challenging (Geber, 1995; Leach and Liu, 2003).

A second major model for training program evaluation is ROI, now often included in training evaluation models as the fifth level of evaluation (Phillips, 1994, 1997). While Kirkpatrick's Level 4 includes measures of the *effectiveness* of training, ROI attempts to assess the *efficiency* of training. ROI is a type of cost-benefit analysis intended to show the relationship between the resources devoted to the training program and the outcomes that result. It requires quantitative measurement of both costs and benefits, which typically proves methodologically challenging. Calculating costs involves not only determining direct costs, such as materials, travel, the training site, meals, equipment, trainers' salaries, and so on, but also accounting for indirect costs, such as participant salaries and lost productivity. Determining benefits requires measuring the difference in work performance or outcomes due to the training (changes in clinical outcomes, medical errors, or patient safety, for example), the monetary value of that performance or outcome, and the expected duration of the training effect—none of which is trivial to determine (Wagner and Weigand, 2004). Phillips (1996a, 1996b) acknowledges multiple challenges in terms of sampling, statistical analysis, the assignment of monetary value to benefits, and so on, though he ultimately argues that such problems can be solved and that ROI evaluation is worthwhile.

While evaluation may become more important and meaningful as the trainee progresses from Level 1 to Level 5, it also becomes more complicated and expensive to implement. Indeed, having trainees fill out evaluation forms is significantly less costly, in terms of both time and money, than developing and administering valid assessments of learning or observing trainee behavior on the job. Furthermore, as we briefly alluded to in describing each level of evaluation, changes in behavior are more difficult to attribute to training than changes in learning, and changes in organization-level outcomes are influenced by an even wider range of extraneous factors, making the measurement and attribution of changes more methodologically challenging at higher levels. As a result, even best-practice organizations tend to use higher-level evaluation only selectively, targeting programs for more rigorous scrutiny based on their cost, strategic importance, or other factors (Dixon, 1996). Phillips and Phillips (2002) suggest the goal of evaluating 100 percent of programs at Level 1, 60 percent at Level 2, 30 percent at Level 3, 10 percent at Level 4, and 5 percent at Level 5; the GAO presents this as an example gradation that an agency could follow when deciding among the various levels of evaluation.

Implications for METC

This chapter examined research and evaluation activities in institutions with missions similar to that of METC—in particular, corporate universities; DMETA, METC's counterpart in the UK; and other federal agencies. Evaluation of training programs to measure their impact on individual and organizational performance and to use the results for organizational and training improvement is central to these organizations. To transform itself into a high-performing, best-practice training institution, it would behoove METC to follow their example. Quite apart from these considerations, given the federal government's ongoing and increasing emphasis on performance measurement and accountability, METC needs to develop research and evaluation capabilities and put in place data systems that can collect a variety of data from multiple sources to prove its "value added" to the mission of the MHS and DoD and its careful stewardship of public resources. To this end, the GAO's framework could help guide the training and development process, especially the evaluation component. The experience and lessons learned from other agencies could be very helpful in the initial stages. The VHA has paid significant attention to evaluation, performance measurement, and organizational improvement, and we believe that METC could benefit from developing a closer collaborative relationship with the VHA.

CHAPTER SIX

Conclusions and Recommendations

Pursuant to the BRAC recommendations, METC is being set up to colocate enlisted medical training in the Army, Navy, and Air Force. When it is fully established, it will be responsible for training personnel in more than 100 enlisted medical specialties and will be the world's largest medical education and training institution, with an annual throughput of 24,500 students, an average daily student load of more than 8,000, and a total of 1,400 faculty and staff members. The vision is for METC to become the nation's leading military medical education and training institution, and its stated goals are to capture best practices and achieve efficiencies in training, i.e., to transform itself into a high-performing "learning" organization.

As part of a larger project, we were asked to examine the need to establish a research and evaluation capability within METC. The study focused on two major research questions:

1. Does METC need a research and evaluation capability?
2. What lessons can be learned from institutions with missions similar to that of METC in terms of research and evaluation activities and the structure and scope of an OIR?

Does METC Need a Research and Evaluation Capability?

The answer to this question is an unequivocal "yes." METC does need a research and evaluation capability to further its long-term goals of becoming a high-performing learning organization and an accredited institution of higher education.

Becoming a High-Performing Organization

Our review showed that high-performing organizations typically adopt models of organizational improvement to guide their strategic efforts and are focused on achieving results and outcomes. Furthermore, "to sustain a focus on results, high-performing organizations continuously assess and benchmark performance and efforts to improve performance" (GAO, 2004b, p. 7). Thus, to support its goal of becoming a high-performing organization, METC will need to develop and sustain the capability to collect, organize, analyze, and use data on a variety of processes and outcomes to support innovation and performance excellence.

Becoming an Accredited Institution

Accreditation bodies are increasingly requiring programs and institutions to develop and implement quality-improvement plans and learning objectives and to provide credible evidence of the value added to student learning and subsequent workforce outcomes. The standards of the various accrediting organizations also specify a variety of quality indicators to be used for assessment and evaluation of occupational education programs, including (among others) graduation or completion rate, employment or placement rate, pass rate on professional licensure exams, employer satisfaction, participant satisfaction, and assessment of occupational skills and knowledge. Notably, several of these indicators require follow-up with program graduates and supervisors. Should METC seek accreditation in the future, it will need a research and evaluation capability to meet the accreditation requirement for institutional improvement plans, embedded assessment, and tracking of a variety of indicators.

What Lessons Can Be Learned from Institutions with Similar Missions?

Insights from Community Colleges and Four-Year Institutions

OIRs in higher-education institutions appear to have a range of functions: data management, internal reporting, external reporting, accreditation, and strategic planning, to name a few. Respondents particularly stressed the importance of organizing data collection and management, delineating common terminology and data definitions, and establishing a centralized data warehouse. The majority of institutions reported conducting periodic surveys of students and faculty, including entry and exit student surveys, student satisfaction surveys, and evaluations of courses and instruction. A few institutions (generally, the four-year colleges and larger community colleges) reported participating in internal research and evaluations of programs or initiatives.

Insights from Corporate Universities

Our review of the literature on corporate universities revealed two important themes. First, although corporate universities differ in scope and function, measurement and evaluation of program effectiveness is always a key component, and corporate training leaders devote significant resources and attention to evaluation. Second, best-practice organizations build evaluation into training programs early by devoting considerable attention to evaluation issues in the program development and planning phase. Third, best-practice organizations emphasize a focus on the customer in their evaluation efforts. Evaluators consult with customers—broadly construed—to determine their requirements are and to learn what standards to set and what to measure (Dixon, 1996). Fourth, evaluation in best-practice organizations is focused not simply on program improvement but on broader organizational improvement as well. Thus, evaluations are designed and implemented with strategic organizational goals in mind.

Insights from the Defence Medical Education and Training Agency

DMETA's approach to training emphasizes continuous evaluation throughout the entire training and development cycle: needs analysis, design and development, delivery, and validation. All training is evaluated to measure the immediate reaction of the individual and the learning transfer achieved by the training activity (stages 1 and 2 in commonly accepted evaluation models). DMETA has been proactive in coordinating higher levels of evaluation, the responsibility of the individual services, to validate changes in the behavior of the individual as a result of the training activity; how well the enhancement of knowledge, skills, or attitudes has prepared an individual for his or her role; and the contribution of training to the achievement of business or operational goals. In addition, DMETA collects data and reports annually on several performance indicators that are part of the Defence Balanced Scorecard.

Insights from Federal Agencies

In 2004, the GAO reported on several federal agencies' experiences and lessons learned regarding designing effective training and development programs, noting that (1) evaluation of training was a key component of the training process, and (2) the agencies had begun to use more comprehensive and sophisticated techniques to assess the extent to which training and development programs increased employees' knowledge and skills and enhanced individual and organizational performance. These techniques included pre- and post-testing, tracking changes in individual and program performance, and some limited use of ROI analyses. Our case study of the VHA (see Kirby et al., 2010) showed that, over the past several years, the VHA has spent considerable time and effort transforming itself into a high-performing learning organization, leveraging its NCOD, a central office that measures and monitors the organizational health of the VHA. In addition, it has strongly embraced continuous assessment, feedback, and redesign for all VHA training and development programs and invested considerable resources in evaluation, performance measurement, and metrics for organizational improvement.

The GAO outlined a strategic framework for designing and implementing effective training and development programs that highlights the importance of integrating evaluation at each step of the process, because agencies need to be able to demonstrate how these efforts help develop employees and improve the agencies' performance.

Recommendations for METC

There is a clear need for a research and evaluation capability within METC that can further its current goal of becoming a high-performing organization and its future goal of being accredited. Such a capability can also help address the federal government's increasing need to measure performance and cost-effectiveness and to provide evidence of the value added by training. Typically, colleges house this type of capability within an OIR, and this requires defining the structure and scope of such an office. Our interviews and literature reviews point to some useful recommendations in this regard.

Structure and Governance

In terms of structure, governance, and staffing, METC would benefit from the following guidance in establishing its OIR:

- Position the METC OIR so that it reports to senior leadership and its director is part of the senior management team. This arrangement would help ensure that the office is taken seriously and that the director has credibility and the authority to access the needed data.
- Ensure that the office is adequately staffed and that the staff have a mix of skills, including technical skills (e.g., statistics, information technology, programming), as well as broader enterprise knowledge and communication and interpersonal skills—particularly the ability to convey the meaning of the data collected on training and development activities. Staffing in OIRs in the larger community colleges and four-year institutions tended to range from four to 14 full-time staff members; size is obviously a function of the scope of the office.

- Collaborate with other METC departments, participate in institutional committees, and extend opportunities for all concerned stakeholders to provide input into the process and gain buy-in.
- Encourage OIR staff to participate in professional associations and networks to learn about best practices and to foster personal and professional growth. In addition, ensure that the OIR director develops collaborative relationships with community colleges, corporate universities, other federal agencies (such as the VHA), and DMETA to learn about best practices in research and evaluation activities.

OIR Scope

In terms of scope, the following recommendations were relevant to METC's mission:

- Examine METC's vision and goals and map them against the types of data needed to measure progress. Then, examine the institutional structure within METC to delineate the roles and responsibilities of the various offices to avoid both duplication of effort and the overlooking of essential functions.
- Consider the following, among other functions, when defining the scope of the OIR:
  - Build a centralized data warehouse to track students, indicators of student learning, and student progress.
  - Work with the leadership team to collect and report data for METC's balanced scorecard and help translate the results so that they can be used for organizational improvement.
  - Collect, analyze, and report basic data on the institution that might be needed for external reporting.
  - Design and evaluate training programs:
    - o Work with other academic offices responsible for the design and implementation of training to incorporate evaluation from the office's inception.
    - o Examine the full gamut of training programs and determine the types of evaluations that might be appropriate for each. Generally accepted models of evaluation have several

stages that involve increasingly more complex and expensive measures. The office could help determine which programs would warrant the higher and more complex levels of evaluation that would require following up with supervisors and others in the field to determine the impact on performance.
  o Communicate and disseminate results in ways that allow them to be used to improve training.
- Work with program accreditation committees to understand the types of data and reporting required, and ensure that these are feasible.

The roles and responsibilities of the OIR are likely to change over time as it matures, but it is important to lay the groundwork now and ensure that these functions are housed somewhere within METC, either in the OIR or in other offices. Perhaps the most immediate and important of these functions is to be proactive: designing a centralized warehouse for data with carefully defined and consistent data elements and data sources, clearly identifying the rationale and responsibility for data collection. The database should be designed to be flexible and adaptable so that it can easily respond to changing and additional demands as METC becomes more established and the scope of the OIR expands. Recognizing the centrality of research and evaluation activities by establishing an OIR under the direction of an experienced institutional researcher is an important first step to becoming a high-performing, results-driven organization.

The Malcolm Baldrige National Quality Award Program: Education Criteria for Performance Excellence and Framework

This appendix first describes the core values and concepts underlying the Baldrige Education Criteria for Performance Excellence and then presents the seven-part framework that constitutes the Baldrige model of organizational improvement.

Education Criteria for Performance Excellence

The Baldrige program posits that the following core values and concepts characterize high-performing organizations.

Visionary Leadership

The organization's senior leaders should set the direction and create a student-focused, learning-oriented climate; adopt and communicate clear and visible values; and set high expectations that balance the needs of all the stakeholders. Leaders need to ensure that strategies, systems, and methods for achieving performance excellence are in place. "Senior leaders should inspire and encourage [the] entire workforce to contribute, to develop and learn, to be innovative, and to embrace change" (Baldrige National Quality Program, 2009, p. 51). In addition, they need to serve as role models "through their ethical behavior and their personal involvement in planning, communicating, coaching the workforce, developing future leaders, reviewing organizational performance, and recognizing members of [the] workforce" (Baldrige National Quality Program, 2009, p. 51).

Learning-Centered Education

Students bring to training different backgrounds, needs, and levels of preparation and should be provided with a variety of avenues for success. A learning-centered organization needs to understand these requirements and translate them into appropriate curricula and learning experiences, focusing on active learning and development of problem-solving skills. "Learning-centered education is a strategic concept that demands constant sensitivity to changing and emerging student, stakeholder, and market requirements and to the factors that drive student learning, satisfaction, and persistence" (Baldrige National Quality Program, 2009, p. 52).

Key characteristics of learning-centered education include (among others) establishing high expectations and standards for all students and incorporating them into assessments, ensuring that faculty members offer support and guidance to help students learn in different ways and at appropriate rates, emphasizing active learning, and using formative assessments to better tailor learning experiences to individual needs and learning styles, as well as summative assessments to measure progress against key standards and norms regarding what students should know and be able to do.

Organizational and Personal Learning

Organizational and personal learning underpin both the core values and the criteria that define performance excellence. Organizational learning is capable of

> (1) enhancing value to students and stakeholders through new and improved programs, offerings, and services; (2) developing new educational opportunities; (3) developing new and improved processes and, as appropriate, business models; (4) reducing errors, variability, waste, and related costs; (5) improving responsiveness and cycle time performance; (6) increasing productivity and effectiveness in the use of all [available] resources; and (7) enhancing your organization's performance in fulfilling its societal responsibilities and its service to your community. (Baldrige National Quality Program, 2009, p. 53)

The Baldrige model emphasizes that learning needs to be embedded in the way in which the organization operates. It cannot be imposed from outside or followed sporadically.

> This means that learning (1) is a regular part of daily work; (2) is practiced at personal, work unit, department, and organizational levels; (3) results in solving problems at their source ("root cause"); (4) is focused on building and sharing knowledge throughout your organization; and (5) is driven by opportunities to effect significant, meaningful change and to innovate. (Baldrige National Quality Program, 2009, p. 53)

Organizations need to invest in personal learning through education, training, and other opportunities for continuing growth and development, including job rotation and increased pay for demonstrated knowledge and skills. Personal learning is important because it results in a more engaged and satisfied workforce, gives faculty and staff a chance to excel, and builds the organization's knowledge assets, allowing it to be more adaptive, innovative, and responsive to the needs of students, stakeholders, and the market.

Valuing the Workforce and Partners

A high-performing organization recognizes that its success depends on an engaged and creative workforce "that benefits from meaningful work, clear organizational direction, and performance accountability and that has a safe, trusting, and cooperative environment" (Baldrige National Quality Program, 2009, p. 53). Organizations show that they value their people by committing to their engagement, satisfaction, and development. The Baldrige model notes major challenges in this area, including providing recognition that goes beyond the regular compensation system and offering development and career progression within the organization.

In addition, organizations need to build internal and external partnerships to better accomplish overall goals. External partnerships (especially strategic alliances) can prove important to an organization's ability to carry out its mission.

Agility

The capacity to respond quickly and flexibly to changing needs and environments is increasingly recognized as essential to succeed in today's globally competitive environment. Educational institutions are expected to respond rapidly to emerging social issues. "A cross-trained and empowered workforce is a vital asset in such a demanding environment" (Baldrige National Quality Program, 2009, p. 54).

Focus on the Future

A strong future orientation and a willingness to make long-term commitments to students and key stakeholders are both important for creating a sustainable organization. Thus, an organization's planning should take into account the factors that might change in the future, such as educational requirements and instructional approaches, workforce development and hiring needs, and technological developments. The model also emphasizes that a major longer-term investment associated with the organization's improvement is

> the investment in creating and sustaining a mission-oriented assessment system focused on learning. . . . In addition, the organization's leaders should be familiar with research findings and practical applications of assessment methods and learning style information. (Baldrige National Quality Program, 2009, p. 55)

Managing for Innovation

Innovation is defined as "making meaningful change to improve an organization's programs, services, processes, operations, and business model, if appropriate, to create new value for the organization's stakeholders" (Baldrige National Quality Program, 2009, p. 55). The Baldrige model notes that innovation is no longer strictly the purview of research and that organizations should be led and managed so that innovation becomes part of the learning culture and is supported by the performance improvement system.

This underscores the importance of encouraging organizational and personal learning so that the organization can rapidly disseminate and capitalize on accumulated knowledge to drive innovation.

Management by Fact

Because this core value is central to the argument that there is a need for a research and evaluation capability within METC, and because this section offers valuable lessons about measuring and analyzing performance, we quote at length from the Baldrige National Quality Program's *2009–2010 Education Criteria for Performance Excellence* (2009, p. 55; emphasis in original).

> Organizations depend on the measurement and analysis of performance. Such measurements should derive from the organization's needs and strategy, and they should provide critical data and information about key processes and results. Many types of data and information are needed for performance management. Performance measurement should focus on student learning, which requires a comprehensive and integrated fact-based system—one that includes input data, environmental data, performance data, comparative/competitive data, workforce data, cost data, process performance, and operational performance measurement. Measurement areas might include students' backgrounds, learning styles, aspirations, academic strengths and weaknesses, educational progress, classroom and program learning, satisfaction with instruction and services, extracurricular activities, dropout/matriculation rates, and postgraduation success. Examples of appropriate data segmentation include, but are not limited to, segmentation by student learning results, student demographics, and workforce groups.
>
> Analysis refers to extracting larger meaning from data and information to support evaluation, decision making, improvement, and innovation. Analysis entails using data to determine trends, projections, and cause and effect that might not otherwise be evident. Analysis supports a variety of purposes, such as planning, reviewing your overall performance, improving operations, accomplishing change management, and comparing your performance with that of organizations providing similar programs and services or with "best practices" benchmarks.
>
> A major consideration in performance improvement and change management involves the selection and use of performance mea-

sures or indicators. *The measures or indicators you select should best represent the factors that lead to improved student, operational, financial, and societal performance. A comprehensive set of measures or indicators tied to student, stakeholder, and organizational performance requirements provides a clear basis for aligning all processes with your organization's goals.* Measures and indicators may need to support decision making in a rapidly changing environment. Through the analysis of data from your tracking processes, your measures or indicators themselves may be evaluated and changed to better support your goals.

Societal Responsibility

The Baldrige model emphasizes the need to recognize the organization's responsibility to the public and to consider societal well-being and benefit. Organizations are encouraged to stress ethical behavior on the part of their leaders and employees; emphasize resource conservation; anticipate adverse impacts that might arise in facilities management, laboratory operations, and transportation; and to go beyond mere compliance with local, state, and federal laws and regulatory requirements.

Focus on Results and Creating Value

An organization's performance metrics should focus on key results. The use of a balanced scorecard type of approach with both leading and lagging performance measures offers "an effective means to communicate short- and longer-term priorities, monitor actual performance, and provide a clear basis for improving results" (Baldrige National Quality Program, 2009, p. 56).

Systems Perspective

As the model notes, the Baldrige education criteria provide a systems perspective for managing the organization and its key processes, helping an organization achieve results and strive for performance excellence. However, success in this arena requires synthesis, alignment, and integration.

Synthesis means looking at your organization as a whole and builds on key educational attributes, including your core competencies, strategic objectives, action plans, and work systems. Alignment means using the key linkages among requirements given in the Baldrige Criteria Categories to ensure consistency of plans, processes, measures, and actions. Integration builds on alignment, so that the individual components of your performance management system operate in a fully interconnected manner and deliver anticipated results. (Baldrige National Quality Program, 2009, p. 56)

The Baldrige Seven-Part Framework

Figure A.1 shows the seven-part framework that constitutes the Baldrige model of organizational improvement. The application for the MBNQA asks institutions to address each of these seven categories. Within each category, a number of questions (not shown) help guide the organization's efforts to use the model for self-assessment or as a first step toward application. We highlight the measurement, analysis, and knowledge management category (box 4 in Figure A.1) as most directly relevant to the purpose of determining whether there is a need for a research and evaluation capability within METC and, if so, what its scope would be.

Organizational Profile

The organizational profile is the starting point for the self-assessment and for filling out the application. It reveals context in which the organization operates and provides an overview of the organization—its operating environment, key relationships, the competitiveness of the environment, its strategic context, and its approach to performance improvement.

The Organizational Profile provides your organization with critical insight into the key internal and external factors that shape your operating environment. These factors, such as the mission, vision, values, core competencies, competitive and collaborative

Figure A.1
Baldrige Education Criteria for Performance Excellence Framework:
A Systems Perspective

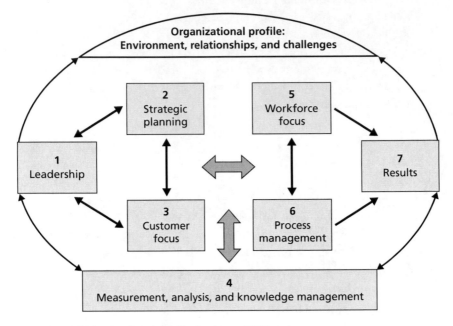

SOURCE: Baldrige National Quality Program, 2009, p. iv.
RAND *MG981-A.1*

environment, and strategic challenges and advantages, impact
the way your organization is run and the decisions you make. As
such, the Organizational Profile helps your organization better
understand the context in which it operates; the key requirements
for current and future organizational success and sustainability;
and the needs, opportunities, and constraints placed on your
organization's management systems. (Baldrige National Quality
Program, 2009, p. 35)

Leadership

The leadership portion of the model addresses how senior leaders'
actions guide and sustain the organization, setting the organization's
vision, values, and performance expectations. Organizations are asked

to pay attention to how senior leaders "communicate with [the] workforce, enhance their personal leadership skills, participate in organizational learning and develop future leaders, measure organizational performance, and create a learning environment that encourages ethical behavior and high performance" (Baldrige National Quality Program, 2009, p. 36). The category also includes the organization's governance system and its legal, ethical, and societal responsibilities.

Strategic Planning

Strategic planning includes how an organization develops a strategy to address its major challenges and leverage its strategic advantages, as well as how it converts its strategic objectives into action plans, how it deploys plans, and how it ensures that adequate resources are available to fulfill the plans' goals. This category also asks how accomplishments are measured and sustained.

Customer Focus

The customer focus portion addresses how the organization seeks to engage students and stakeholders, emphasizing that building these relationships is an important part of a performance excellence strategy. The model points out that balancing the differing needs and expectations of students and stakeholders can prove challenging and suggests that "the voice of the customer" can provide meaningful information that can contribute to the sustainability of the organization.

Measurement, Analysis, and Knowledge Management

In the simplest terms, Category 4 is the "brain center" for the alignment of your organization's programs and offerings with its strategic objectives. Central to such use of data and information are their quality and availability. Furthermore, since information, analysis, and knowledge management might themselves be core competencies that provide an advantage in your market or service environment, this Category also includes such strategic considerations. (Baldrige National Quality Program, 2009, p. 41)

This measurement, analysis, and knowledge management category focuses on two questions: How does the organization measure, analyze, and improve organizational performance, and how does it manage information, organizational knowledge, and information technology? We focus on the first, which asks how the organization selects and uses data and information for performance measurement, analysis, and review in support of organizational planning and performance improvement. The organizational review is intended to cover all areas of performance, including current and future anticipated performance, with the purpose of translating review findings into an action agenda that is sufficiently specific for deployment throughout the organization and to students, key stakeholders, and partners. The guidelines suggest several types of analyses that might help organizations gain an understanding of performance and needed actions. We list a selection here:

> how program, offering, and service improvements correlate with key student and stakeholder indicators, such as student achievement, student and stakeholder satisfaction and retention, and market share
>
> the relationship among student experiences, outcomes, and program completion
>
> the relationship among student experiences, outcomes, and post-program outcomes in peer schools
>
> activity-level cost trends in organizational operations
>
> the relationship between student demographics and outcomes
>
> the percentage of students attaining licenses, industry-recognized certifications, or other professional credentials
>
> cost and financial implications of new educational programs, services, and market entry, and changing educational and operational needs and their impact on organizational sustainability (Baldrige National Quality Program, 2009, pp. 41–42)

The guidelines warn that facts and data alone are not a good basis for setting organizational priorities and that there must be close alignment between analysis and organizational performance review and between analysis and organizational planning to ensure that the data collected are relevant for decisionmaking. In addition,

> [a]ction depends on understanding cause-effect connections among processes and between processes and results or outcomes. . . . Organizations have a critical need to provide an effective analytical basis for decisions, because resources for improvement are limited and cause-effect connections often are unclear. (Baldrige National Quality Program, 2009, p. 42)

Workforce Focus

This category looks at key workforce practices—those directed toward creating and maintaining a high-performance work environment with a strong focus on students and learning. The category addresses how the organization engages, manages, and develops its workforce in an integrated way (i.e., aligned with the organization's strategic objectives and action plans).

Process Management

The process management category looks at how the work of the organization is accomplished: work systems and work process design, key work processes, work process management, work process improvement, and emergency readiness.

Results

This category examines the organization's performance and improvement in six key areas: student learning; customer-focused outcomes; budgetary, financial, and market outcomes; workforce outcomes; process effectiveness; and leadership. The category is intended to provide "real-time" information or measures of progress that can be used to evaluate and improve educational programs, offerings, and services, as well as the organization's processes, in alignment with the overall organizational strategy.

References

ABHES—*see* Accrediting Bureau of Health Education Schools.

Accrediting Bureau of Health Education Schools, homepage, undated. As of August 19, 2010:
http://www.abhes.org/

———, *Accreditation Manual*, 16th ed., Falls Church, Va., 2010. As of August 19, 2010:
http://www.abhes.org/assets/uploads/files/2010-01-084b479cfd2cff9ABHES%20 16th%20Edition%20Manual%202010.pdf

AEA—*see* American Evaluation Association.

AERA—*see* American Educational Research Association.

AIR—*see* Association for Institutional Research.

Air University, "CCAF Accreditation," web page, undated. As of August 19, 2010:
http://www.au.af.mil/au/ccaf/academics/accreditation.asp

Allen, Mark, ed., *The Corporate University Handbook*, New York: AMACOM, 2002.

Allen, Mark, and Philip McGee, "Measurement and Evaluation in Corporate Universities," *New Directions for Institutional Research*, Vol. 124, 2004, pp. 81–92.

Alliger, George M., Scott I. Tannenbaum, Winston Bennett, Jr., Holly Traver, and Allison Shotland, "A Meta-Analysis of the Relations Among Training Criteria," *Personnel Psychology*, Vol. 50, No. 2, June 1997, pp. 341–358.

American Educational Research Association, "About AERA," web page, last updated June 4, 2010. As of August 19, 2010:
http://www.aera.net/AboutAERA.htm

American Evaluation Association, "About Us," web page, undated. As of August 19, 2010:
http://www.eval.org/aboutus/organization/aboutus.asp

ASHE—*see* Association for the Study of Higher Education.

Association for Institutional Research, "Code of Ethics for Institutional Research," brochure, 2002.

Association for the Study of Higher Education, homepage, undated. As of August 19, 2010:
http://www.ashe.ws/

Baldrige National Quality Program, "2005 Award Winner," Richland College profile, Gaithersburg, Md., 2005. As of August 19, 2010:
http://www.baldrige.nist.gov/PDF_files/Richland_College_Profile.pdf

————, *2009–2010 Education Criteria for Performance Excellence*, Gaithersburg, Md.: National Institute of Standards and Technology, 2009. As of August 19, 2010:
http://www.baldrige.nist.gov/Education_Criteria.htm

————, "Why Take the Baldrige Journey?" web page, last updated July 13, 2010a. As of August 19, 2010:
http://www.nist.gov/baldrige/enter/index.cfm

————, "Baldrige Award Recipients' Contacts and Profiles," web page, last updated July 22, 2010b. As of August 19, 2010:
http://www.baldrige.nist.gov/Contacts_Profiles.htm

Barnett, Carol K., *Rethinking Organizational Learning Theories: A Review and Synthesis of the Primary Literature*, unpublished research, Durham, N.H.: Whittemore School of Business and Economics, University of New Hampshire, undated.

Bober, Christopher F., and Kenneth R. Bartlett, "The Utilization of Training Program Evaluation in Corporate Universities," *Human Resource Development Quarterly*, Vol. 15, No. 4, Winter 2004, pp. 363–383.

Camp, Richaurd R., P. Nick Blanchard, and Gregory E. Huszczo, *Toward a More Organizationally Effective Training Strategy and Practice*, Englewood Cliffs, N.J.: Prentice Hall, 1986.

Campion, Michael A., and James E. Campion, "Evaluation of an Interviewee Skills Training Program in a Natural Field Experiment," *Personnel Psychology*, Vol. 40, No. 4, December 1987, pp. 675–691.

Choo, Chun Wei, *The Knowing Organization: How Organizations Use Information to Construct Meaning, Create Knowledge, and Make Decisions*, New York: Oxford University Press, 1998.

Code of Federal Regulations, Title 45, Public Welfare, Department of Health and Human Services, Part 46, Protection of Human Subjects, effective July 14, 2009. As of August 19, 2010:
http://www.hhs.gov/ohrp/documents/OHRPRegulations.pdf

COE—*see* Council on Occupational Accreditation.

Council on Higher Education Accreditation, homepage, undated. As of August 19, 2010:
http://www.chea.org/

Council on Occupational Education, homepage, undated. As of August 19, 2010:
http://www.council.org/

———, *Handbook of Accreditation, 2010 Edition*, Atlanta, Ga., 2010. As of August 19, 2010:
http://www.council.org/files/show/2010%20Handbook%20FINAL%20w%20Covers%202-11-10.pdf

Daft, Richard L., *Organization Theory and Design*, 6th ed., Cincinnati, Ohio: South-Western College Publishing, 1998.

Daft, Richard L., and Norman B. Macintosh, "A Tentative Exploration into the Amount and Equivocality of Information Processing in Organizational Work Units," *Administrative Science Quarterly*, Vol. 26, No. 2, June 1981, pp. 207–224.

Dean, James W., Jr., and Mark P. Sharfman, "The Relationship Between Procedural Rationality and Political Behavior in Strategic Decision Making," *Decision Sciences*, Vol. 24, No. 6, 1993, pp. 1069–1083.

De Gues, Arie P., "Planning as Learning," *Harvard Business Review*, March–April 1988, pp. 70–74.

Defence Medical Education and Training Agency, *Defence Medical Education and Training Agency Framework Document*, London, 2003.

———, *Annual Report 2007/2008*, London: Stationery Office, 2008. As of August 19, 2010:
http://www.official-documents.gov.uk/document/hc0708/hc08/0834/0834.pdf

Dixon, Nancy M., "New Routes to Evaluation," *Training and Development*, May 1996, pp. 82–85.

DMETA—*see* Defence Medical Education and Training Agency.

Drucker, Peter, "Knowledge-Worker Productivity: The Biggest Challenge," *California Management Review*, Vol. 41, No. 2, Winter 1999, pp. 79–94.

Feldman, Martha S., and James G. March, "Information in Organizations as Signal and Symbol," *Administrative Science Quarterly*, Vol. 26, No. 2, June 1981, pp. 171–186.

GAO—*see* U.S. General Accounting Office.

Garvin, David A., Amy C. Edmondson, and Francesca Gino, "Is Yours a Learning Organization?" *Harvard Business Review*, March 2008, pp. 109–116.

Geber, Beverly, "Does Your Training Make a Difference? Prove It!" *Training*, Vol. 32, No. 3, March 1995, pp. 27–34.

Ghobadian, Abby, and Hong Seng Woo, "Characteristics, Benefits, and Shortcomings of Four Major Quality Awards," *International Journal Quality and Reliability Management*, Vol. 13, No. 2, 1996, pp. 10–44.

Honeycutt, Earl D., and Thomas H. Stevenson, "Evaluating Sales Training Programs," *Industrial Marketing Management*, Vol. 18, No. 3, August 1989, pp. 215–222.

Huber, George, "A Theory of the Effects of Advanced Information Technologies on Organizational Design, Intelligence, and Decision Making," *Academy of Management Review*, Vol. 15, No. 1, January 1990, pp. 47–71.

Kirby, Sheila Nataraj, "Malcolm Baldrige National Quality Award Program," in Brian Stecher and Sheila Nataraj Kirby, eds., *Organizational Improvement and Accountability: Lessons for Education from Other Sectors*, Santa Monica, Calif.: RAND Corporation, MG-136-WFHF, 2004, pp. 11–33. As of August 19, 2010: http://www.rand.org/pubs/monographs/MG136/

Kirby, Sheila Nataraj, Julie A. Marsh, Jennifer Sloan McCombs, Harry J. Thie, Nailing Xia, and Jerry M. Sollinger, *Developing Military Health Care Leaders: Insights from the Military, Civilian, and Government Sectors*, Santa Monica, Calif.: RAND Corporation, MG-967-OSD, 2010. As of October 2010: http://www.rand.org/pubs/monographs/MG967/

Kirby, Sheila Nataraj, and Harry J. Thie, *Qualifying Military Health Care Officers as "Joint": Weighing the Pros and Cons*, Santa Monica, Calif.: RAND Corporation, MG-775-OSD, 2009. As of August 19, 2010: http://www.rand.org/pubs/monographs/MG775/

Kirkpatrick, Donald L., "Techniques for Evaluating Training Programs," *Journal of the American Society for Training and Development*, Vol. 13, No. 11, 1959, pp. 3–9.

Leach, Mark P., and Annie H. Liu, "Investigating Interrelationships Among Sales Training Evaluation Methods," *Journal of Personal Selling and Sales Management*, Vol. 23, No. 4, Fall 2003, pp. 327–339.

Lipshitz, Raanan, Micha Popper, and Victor J. Friedman, "A Multifacet Model of Organizational Learning," *Journal of Applied Behavioral Science*, Vol. 38, No. 1, March 2002, pp. 78–98.

Lupton, Robert A., John E. Weiss, and Robin T. Peterson, "Sales Training Evaluation Model (STEM): A Conceptual Framework," *Industrial Marketing Management*, Vol. 28, No. 1, January 1999, pp. 73–84.

Mann, Sandi, and Ivan T. Robertson, "What Should Training Evaluations Evaluate?" *Journal of European Industrial Training*, Vol. 20, No. 9, 1996, pp. 14–21.

Markus, M. Lynne, "Power, Politics, and MIS Implementation," *Communications of the ACM*, Vol. 26, No. 6, June 1983, pp. 430–444.

Meister, Jeanne C., *Corporate Quality Universities: Lessons in Building a World-Class Work Force*, Alexandria, Va.: American Society for Training and Development, 1994.

Morest, Vanessa Smith, and Davis Jenkins, *Institutional Research and the Culture of Evidence at Community Colleges*, New York: Community College Research Center, Teachers College, Columbia University, April 2007.

National Institute of Standards and Technology, "Malcolm Baldrige National Quality Award," web page, last updated December 7, 2009. As of August 19, 2010: http://www.nist.gov/public_affairs/factsheet/mbnqa.cfm

NIST—*see* National Institute of Standards and Technology.

Nonaka, Ikujiro, "The Knowledge-Creating Company," *Harvard Business Review*, Vol. 69, No. 6, November–December 1991, pp. 96–104.

Nonaka, Ikujiro, and Georg von Krogh, "Tacit Knowledge and Knowledge Conversion: Controversy and Advancement in Organizational Knowledge Creation Theory," *Organization Science*, Vol. 20, No. 3, May–June 2009, pp. 635–652.

Office of Management and Budget, *Analytical Perspectives: Budget of the U.S. Government, Fiscal Year 2011*, Washington, D.C., 2010. As of August 19, 2010: http://www.whitehouse.gov/omb/budget/Analytical_Perspectives/.

Ostrom, Elinor, *Governing the Commons: The Evolution of Institutions for Collective Action*, New York: Cambridge University Press, 1990.

Phillips, Jack J., *Measuring Return on Investment*, Vol. 1, Alexandria, Va.: American Society for Training and Development, 1994.

———, "ROI: The Search for Best Practices," *Training and Development*, Vol. 50, No. 2, February 1996a, pp. 42–47.

———, "Was It the Training?" *Training and Development*, Vol. 50, No. 3, March 1996b, pp. 28–32.

———, *Return on Investment in Training and Performance Improvement Programs*, Boston, Mass.: Butterworth-Heinemann, 1997.

Phillips, Patricia Pulliam, and Jack J. Phillips, "The Public Sector Challenge: Developing a Credible ROI Process," in Jack J. Phillips and Patricia Pulliam Phillips, eds., *Measuring ROI in the Public Sector*, Alexandria, Virginia: American Society for Training and Development, 2002, pp. 1–32.

Public Law 100-107, The Malcolm Baldrige National Quality Improvement Act of 1987, August 20, 1987.

Public Law 105-244, 1998 Amendments to the Higher Education Act of 1965, October 7, 1998.

Richland College, *2005 Malcolm Baldrige National Quality Award Application*, Dallas, Tex., 2005. As of August 19, 2010:
http://www.baldrige.nist.gov/PDF_files/Richland_College_Application_Summary.pdf

SACS—*see* Southern Association of Colleges and Schools Commission on Colleges.

Schein, Edgar H., "How Can Organizations Learn Faster? The Challenge of Entering the Green Room," *Sloan Management Review*, Vol. 32, No. 2, Winter 1993.

Senge, Peter M., *The Fifth Discipline: The Art and Practice of the Learning Organization*, New York: Doubleday, 1990a.

———, "The Leader's New Work: Building Learning Organizations," *Sloan Management Review*, Vol. 32, No. 1, Fall 1990b.

Serenko, Alexander, Nick Bontis, and Timothy Hardie, "Organizational Size and Knowledge Flow," *Journal of Intellectual Capital*, Vol. 8, No. 4, 2007, pp. 610–627.

Simon, Herbert A., "Bounded Rationality and Organizational Learning," *Organization Science*, Vol. 2, No. 1, February 1991, pp. 125–134.

Southern Association of Colleges and Schools Commission on Colleges, homepage, undated. As of August 19, 2010:
http://www.sacscoc.org/

———, *Resource Manual for the Principles of Accreditation: Foundations for Quality Enhancement*, Decatur, Ga., 2005. As of August 19, 2010:
http://www.sacscoc.org/pdf/handbooks/Exhibit%2031.Resource%20Manual.pdf

———, *The Principles of Accreditation: Foundations for Quality Enhancement*, Decatur, Ga., 2009a. As of August 19, 2010:
http://www.sacscoc.org/pdf/2010principlesofacreditation.pdf

———, *Handbook for Institutions Seeking Reaffirmation*, Decatur, Ga., December 2009b. As of August 19, 2010:
http://www.sacscoc.org/pdf/081705/Handbook%20for%20Institutions%20seeking%20reaffirmation.pdf

———, "Member, Candidate and Applicant List," Decatur, Ga., July 2010. As of August 19, 2010:
http://www.sacscoc.org/pdf/webmemlist.pdf

Thie, Harry J., Sheila Nataraj Kirby, Adam C. Resnick, Thomas Manacapilli, Daniel Gershwin, Andrew Baxter, and Roland J. Yardley, *Enhancing Interoperability Among Enlisted Medical Personnel: A Case Study of Military Surgical Technologists*, Santa Monica, Calif.: RAND Corporation, MG-774-OSD, 2009. As of August 19, 2010:
http://www.rand.org/pubs/monographs/MG774/

Turban, Efraim, Ephraim R. McLean, and James C. Wetherbe, *Information Technology for Management: Improving Quality and Productivity*, New York: Wiley, 1996.

UK Ministry of Defence, Director General, Training and Education, *The Defence Systems Approach to Training Quality Standard*, March 7, 2003.

———, *Ministry of Defense Annual Reports and Accounts, 2004–05*, London: Stationery Office, October 28, 2005. As of August 19, 2010: http://www.mod.uk/NR/rdonlyres/77D6FC7B-7514-4B49-A775-0FDEACF6363 1/0/mod_ara0405_intro.pdf

U.S. Department of Veterans Affairs, *Veterans Health Administration Workforce Succession Strategic Plan, FY 2008–2012*, Washington, D.C., October 2007.

———, *Veterans Health Administration Workforce Succession Strategic Plan*, Washington, D.C., 2009.

U.S. General Accounting Office, *Human Capital: Selected Agencies' Experiences and Lessons Learned in Designing Training and Development Programs*, Washington, D.C., GAO-04-291, January 2004a.

———, *Comptroller General's Forum: High-Performing Organizations*, Washington, D.C., GAO-04-343SP, February 2004b.

———, *Human Capital: A Guide for Assessing Strategic Training and Development Efforts in the Federal Government*, Washington, D.C., GAO-04-546G, March 2004c.

VA—*see* U.S. Department of Veterans Affairs.

Wagner, Richard J., and Robert J. Weigand, "Can the Value of Training Be Measured? A Simplified Approach to Evaluating Training," *Health Care Manager*, Vol. 23, No. 1, January–March 2004, pp. 71–77.

Wang, Greg G., and Dean R. Spitzer, "Human Resource Development Measurement and Evaluation: Looking Back and Moving Forward," *Advances in Developing Human Resources*, Vol. 7, No. 1, February 2005, pp. 5–15.

Walker, David M., "The Role of GAO and Other Government Auditors in the 21st Century," speech, Forum of Government Auditors, Providence, R.I., May 20, 2002. As of August 19, 2010: http://www.gao.gov/cghome/2002/14thbf.html

Warr, Peter B., and David Bunce, "Trainee Characteristics and the Outcomes of Open Learning," *Personnel Psychology*, Vol. 48, No. 2, June 1995, pp. 347–375.

Watson, Scott C., "Five Easy Pieces to Performance Measurement," *Training and Development*, Vol. 52, No. 5, May 1998, pp. 44–49.

Weiss, Carol H., "Ideology, Interests, and Information," in Daniel Callahan and Bruce Jennings, eds., *The Social Sciences and Policy Analysis*, New York: Plenum Press, 1983, pp. 224–250.